PERINATAL MORTALITY

Edited by **Oliver C. Ezechi**
and **Karen Odberg-Petterson**

Perinatal Mortality
Edited by Oliver C. Ezechi and Karen Odberg-Petterson

Published by InTech

Janeza Trdine 9, 51000 Rijeka, Croatia

Publishing Process Manager Romina Skomersic

Technical Editor Teodora Smiljanic

Cover Designer InTech Design Team

Additional hard copies can be obtained from orders@intechopen.com

Perinatal Mortality, Edited by Oliver C. Ezechi and Karen Odberg-Petterson
p. cm.
ISBN 978-953-51-0659-3

For EU product safety concerns:
IN TECH d.o.o., Prolaz Marije Krucifikse Kozulić 3, 51000 Rijeka, Croatia,
info@intechopen.com or visit our website at intechopen.com.

Meet the editors

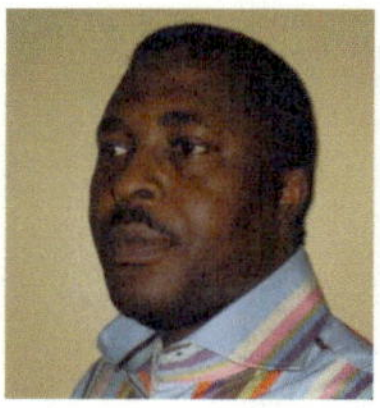

Dr Oliver C. Ezechi is a trained Obstetrician and Gynaecologist, and a Chief Research Fellow at the Nigerian Institute of Medical Research Lagos, Nigeria, where he coordinates the Maternal, Reproductive and Child Health Research programmes, as well as heads the Clinical Sciences Division. He holds additional qualifications and expertise in public health and health services administration. Dr Ezechi has over 20 years of experience in maternal and reproductive health, including 11 years of research and teaching. He has travelled widely to study and acquaint himself with maternal and reproductive health development in different countries. He has to his credit more than 50 publications in the areas of maternal and reproductive health, published in national and international peer-reviewed journals.

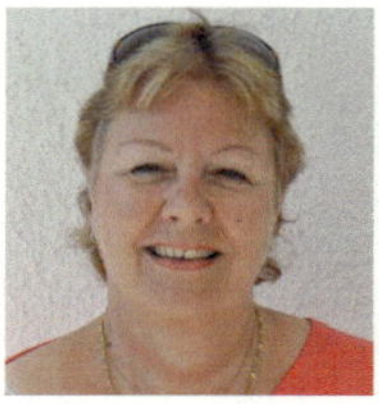

Dr Karen Odberg Pettersson, MNsc, MPH, Med.Dr, is by profession a registered nurse and midwife tutor and currently employed as a researcher at the Faculty of Medicine at Lund University; Div. of Social Medicine and Global Health in Malmö. Dr Odberg Pettersson has more than 30 years of international experience in maternal and neonatal health, including program implementation, consultation and teaching & curriculum development. Besides continued international research, her focus for the last 5 years has been on advanced training in sexual and reproductive health and rights, an international program for teams of obstetricians and midwives. The many travels to teams from South East Asia, Africa, Central Asia and East Europe to supervise projects which are part of this training, have resulted with the honorary title "globetrotter in maternal health".

Contents

Preface

It gives us great pleasure to present the book "Perinatal Mortality". We have taken great pain to ensure quality and that current articles on the subject of perinatology are included. A variety of subjects ranging from global overview of perinatal mortality, trends in low income countries, effect of some medical disorders on perinatal morbidity and mortality, strategies for its prevention and control, and future trends were covered by experts in the field.

The information presented in the book will, hopefully, benefit not only professionals in the perinatal medicine, but also other clinicians, scientists and students who would like to improve and expand their understanding of perinatal mortality and the best strategies to its reduction, both in low and high income countries.

I thank all the contributing authors who have generously given their expertise and time to make this book a reality. They kept the deadline despite their very busy and tight schedules. This show of scholarship is greatly appreciated. To colleagues who assisted with peer-review of the chapters, we cannot thank you enough. We have to respect your wish of remaining unanimous, otherwise we would have preferred to document your names in this book for posterity.

Technical assistance provided by InTech Editorial Office during the production of the book is gratefully acknowledged.

Oliver C. Ezechi
Chief Research Fellow & Consultant Obstetrician and Gynaecologist,
Division of Clinical Sciences, Nigerian Institute of Medical Research (NIMR),
Lagos,
Nigeria

Karen Odberg-Pettersson
Faculty of Medicine, Lund University,
Sweden

1

Overview of Global Perinatal Mortality

Oliver C. Ezechi and Agatha N. David
Division of Clinical Sciences,
Maternal, Reproductive and Child Health Research Programme,
Nigerian Institute of Medical Research,
Lagos

1. Introduction

Perinatal mortality refers to the death of a fetus or neonate and is the basis to calculate the perinatal mortality rate. The perinatal period is the most vulnerable period in the life of an individual and the rate of death during this period is higher than at any other period of life. Deaths during this short period equal the rate of death over the next forty year period. Social, cultural, environmental and genetic factors all play vital roles in determining the outcome of this period of life.

Perinatal mortality is at an unacceptably high level in low income countries, especially those in sub-Saharan Africa and south central Asia [1]. Recent estimates show that the perinatal mortality rate in high income countries of the world is about 10 per 1000 live births compared with 50 per 1000 live births in low income countries [2]. These figures are particularly troubling because the perinatal mortality rate is a key indicator of the health status of a community. Specifically, it reflects the quality of prenatal, delivery and early infant care practices available in any setting. It is also a major contributor to overall under-five mortality [1].

Reducing the 1990 childhood mortality levels by two-thirds by the year 2015 is one of the Millennium Development Goals (MDG-4) set by the United Nations. Recent evidence shows that perinatal mortality accounts for about 40% of infant mortality globally (Figure 1). In addition 75% of all neonatal deaths occur during the perinatal period. It is therefore obvious that MDG-4 cannot be achieved without substantially reducing these perinatal deaths most especially in the high burden countries of south central Asia and sub Saharan Africa. [3, 4].

While substantial gains have been made in the reduction of infant and under5 mortality rates (IMR and U5MR), same cannot be said for perinatal and neonatal mortality rates. As a result of this disparity, neonatal mortality now accounts for a greater proportion of IMR. Neonatal mortality was responsible for 27% of IMR globally in 1970 but accounted for 41% of IMR in 2010 [5]. In countries with low IMR and U5MR, the NMR accounts for an even higher proportion of IMR [1-5].

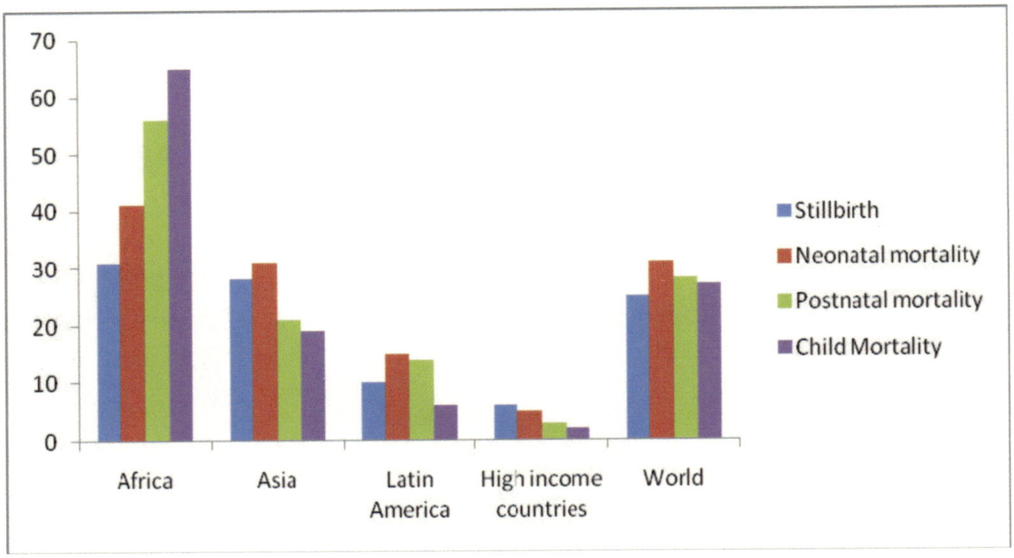

Fig. 1. Child mortality and stillbirth rates in 2000 - adapted from WHO 2005[1]

While perinatal mortality rate is a useful indicator of the quality of antenatal and perinatal care, its wholesale application in international comparisons can be misleading if a number of factors and important determinants that need to be assessed separately before reaching conclusions about quality-of-care issues are not taken into consideration [6].

This chapter provides a general overview of perinatal mortality. It will address the burden of perinatal mortality and its contribution to global childhood deaths. The relationship between quality of antenatal and perinatal care and risk factors for perinatal mortality, and how these lead to the perinatal mortality rate will be discussed. Finally evidence based strategies for reduction and prevention of perinatal mortality and future thrust will be highlighted.

2. Definition of terms

Neonatal Period: The first 28 days of post natal life is the neonatal period. It is subdivided into the immediate (first 24hours), early (first 7 days) and late (8-28 days) neonatal periods.

Perinatal Period: This is the period from the age of viability of the fetus to the first 7 days of postnatal life.

Live birth: A product of conception which, after complete extraction from its mother, shows signs of life such as breathing, beating of the heart, umbilical cord pulsation or spontaneous movement of voluntary muscles regardless of gestational age and whether the cord has been cut or the placenta has been extracted or not.

Stillbirth: Still birth refers to fetal mortality or death. According to WHO, stillbirth is the birth of a baby with a birth weight of 500 g or more, 22 or more completed weeks of gestation, or a body length of 25 cm or more, who died before or during labour and birth. For international comparisons, WHO recommends reporting of stillbirths with birth weight of 1000 g or more, 28 weeks' gestation or more, or a body length of 35 cm or more [4].

Neonatal mortality: Neonatal mortality (NM) refers to neonatal death. It is the death of a new born within the first 28 days of life. It can also be divided into death of a live-born baby within the first seven days of life (early neonatal mortality-ENM) and death after 7 days until 28th day of life (late neonatal mortality-LNM).

$$NM = ENM + LNM$$

Perinatal Mortality: Perinatal mortality (PM) refers to the death of a fetus after the age of viability, until the 7th day of life. It equals the sum of still birth and early neonatal death. PM = SB + ENM

Neonatal Mortality Rate: Neonatal mortality rate (NMR) is the number of deaths which occur in the first 28 days of life over the total number of live births in a given locality over a given time period divided by 1000. It is usually expressed as *number of deaths per 1000 live births.*

Still birth rate: Still birth rate (SBR) is the number of fetal loss prior to or during labour i.e. babies born dead over the total number of births in a given period and *is expressed as still births per thousand births.*

3. Perinatal mortality rate

Varying definitions have been applied to perinatal mortality rate. While some definitions are more inclusive and encompass infant deaths at age of less than 28 days of age and fetal deaths of 20 or more weeks gestation, the more conservative definition that only includes infant deaths of less than seven days of age and fetal deaths of 28 or more weeks gestation is preferred for international and region-to-region comparisons due to differences among countries/regions in completeness of reporting of fetal deaths of 20-27 weeks gestation.

Perinatal mortality rate (PNMR) is the total number of still births plus deaths in the first 7 days of postnatal life in a given time period over the total number of births multiplied by a thousand and is expressed *as number of deaths per 1000 births.* It is usually reported on an annual basis. It is a major marker to assess the quality of health care delivery in a community. Comparisons between regions/countries may be hampered by varying definitions, registration bias, and differences in the underlying risks of the populations.

$$\text{PNMR} = \left[\frac{(\text{Number of stillbirth} + \text{Number of early neonatal deaths})}{(\text{Number of live births} + \text{Number of stillbirth})}\right] \text{X } 1{,}000$$

4. Epidemiology

Globally about 3 million of the 130 million babies born every year die in the first 4 weeks of life and another 2.65 million die even before their first breath of life, most often in the last 12 weeks of pregnancy [7]. Low income and middle income countries account for over 99% of these perinatal deaths. Unfortunately most of these fetuses and infants are unnamed and unrecorded, indicating the perceived inevitability of their deaths, and thus unaccounted for [5]. It is therefore not suprising that the reported mortality figures are only estimates and may just be a tip of the iceberg.

Three-quarters of neonatal deaths occur in the first week with the highest risk of death on the first day of life (figure 2).

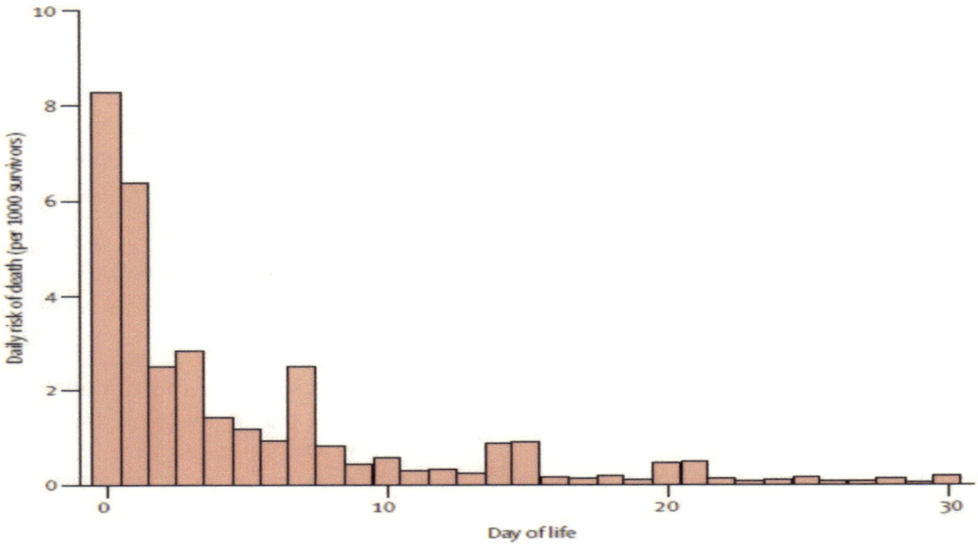

Fig. 2. Daily risk of death during first month of life (adapted from Lawn JE et al)]6]

While the south central Asian countries account for the highest numbers of neonatal deaths, the countries with highest rates are generally in sub-Saharan Africa. Ten countries account for 75% of all neonatal deaths, with India, China, Pakistan and Nigeria leading the pack (Table 1). Over 82% of all neonatal deaths occurs in South central Asia and sub-Saharan with sub-regional variations.

Country	Number of neonatal (1000s)	Percentage of global neonatal deaths (n=3 99 million)	NMR (per 1000 live births)
India	1098	27%	43
China	416	10%	21
Pakistan	298	7%	57
Nigeria	247	6%	53
Bangladesh	153	4%	36
Ethiopia	147	4%	51
Democratic Republic of Congo	116	3%	47
Indonesia	82	2%	18
Afghanistan	63	2%	60
United Republic of Tanzania	62	2%	43
Total	2682	67%	

Table 1. Countries with largest number of global neonatal mortality
(adapted from Lawn JE) [6]

Though most of the countries in south central Asia and sub Saharan African have made little progress in reducing perinatal deaths in the past decade, it is important to note that some progress has been made [9]. During the past decade, China has dropped from the second to fourth highest burden of stillbirths because of a rapid reduction in stillbirth rate and a reduced total fertility rate. Nigeria has moved up to the second highest as the national stillbirth rate and total fertility rate remain high [6].

There are also major differences in perinatal mortality rates within countries and regions . In India and Nigeria large variations exist between rural and urban communities. The rates in rural northern communities in Nigeria are higher than those for urban hospitals in southern Nigeria [6,10,11]. In high income countries and Latin America, rates are higher in urban than rural communities [65]. However two-thirds of all stillbirths occur in rural communities and families.

Unlike early neonatal deaths, stillbirths are not just a low-income country problem. Rates in the UK and USA have decreased by only 1% per year for the past 15 years and stillbirths now account for two-thirds of perinatal deaths in the UK [12, 13] .

4.1 Causes and determinants of perinatal mortality

Childhood mortality has been declining globally as a result of socioeconomic development and implementation of child survival interventions, yet approximately 6 million infants die every year before the end of their first week of life. The prevention of perinatal death is greatly dependent on ascertaining the causes of the deaths and the background factors associated with them. Across the globe the causes of perinatal deaths are strikingly similar, although their relative importance varies between countries, regions and income status.

Several important features about perinatal mortality are common globally. The same socioeconomic, biologic and health factors that influence maternal deaths are also at play in causing perinatal deaths and rates. For ease of comprehension, the causes and determinants of perinatal mortality will be discussed under two headings of direct and indirect. It is however important to note that often the causes are characterized by a chain of events leading to death making it impossible to single out one factor as the sole cause of the perinatal death. For example; an unbooked primigravida who presents in the hospital with prolonged labour and arrives the hospital with fetal heart present. Unfortunately the hospital requires a cash deposit to be paid before the woman can be attended to. By the time her relatives are able to make the cash deposit three hours later, the fetal heart has disappeared. What is the cause of still birth in this situation? Is it due to the background factors of unbooked status, primigravida status, late presentation, prolonged labour, phase three delay at the hospital due to hospital policy of user fee charges even in emergency situation, or poverty?. This scenario is a common finding in low income perinatology.

4.2 Direct causes

Causes of neonatal deaths are often difficult to decipher, because most of the births occur outside authorized health facilities unattended by health workers, or because the neonates present with non-specific signs and symptoms. However most neonatal deaths result from complications of preterm birth, asphyxia, birth trauma, infections and severe congenital malformations. The proportion of neonatal death due to each cause differs between areas with high and low perinatal mortality rates. While in high and middle income countries with low rates, preterm births and malformations account for majority of the deaths, in south -central Asia and sub-Saharan Africa with high rates, asphyxia, tetanus, and infections are the leading causes [5].

Estimates from 2008 of the distribution of direct causes of neonatal death, indicate that preterm birth [29.3 %], severe infections (, including sepsis and pneumonia) [25%], tetanus [2.4%], and diarrhoea [2.4%]), and complications of asphyxia (22%) account for most neonatal deaths. Congenital anomalies account for 7.3% of the remaining 19.5% (figure 3).

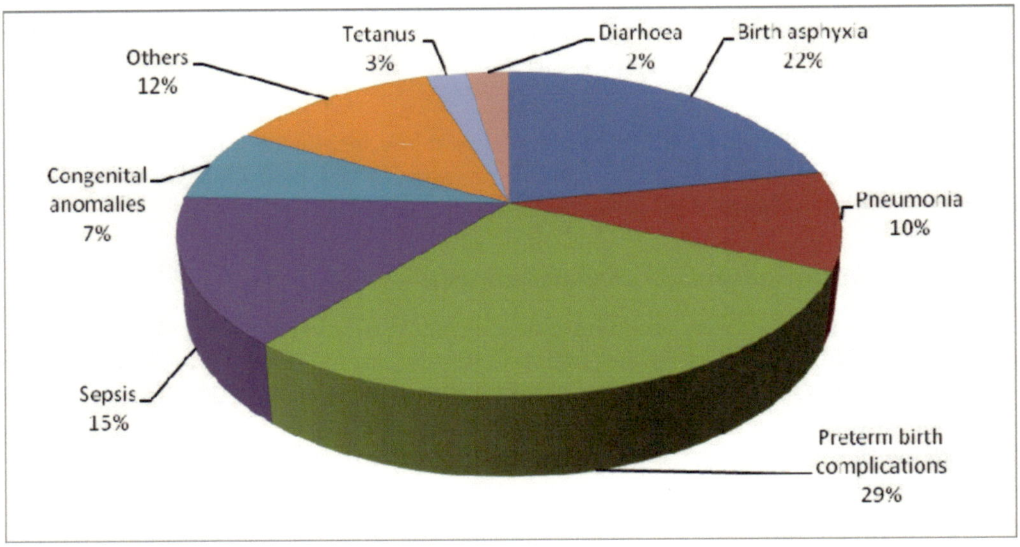

Fig. 3. Causes of neonatal deaths (adapted from Black RE et al 2008) [14].

Low birth weight is associated with the death of many newborn infants, but is not considered a direct cause. The complications stemming from preterm delivery, rather than low birth weight are the direct cause of early neonatal death. Around 15% of newborn infants weigh less than 2500 g, the proportion ranging from 6% in developed countries to more than 30% in some parts of the world [2].

The events leading to the delivery of a baby "still" may occur either before onset of labour (antepartum death) or during labour (intrapartum death). These deaths may be as a result of pregnancy complications or maternal illness. Often no identifiable cause could be found for many antepartum fetal deaths. Complications arising during delivery are the major cause of death among fetuses, who were alive when labour started. Such complications include cord accidents, malpresentation, deep transverse arrest and uterine rupture.

4.3 Indirect causes

Several maternal, obstetric, health system and socioeconomic factors and conditions indirectly contribute to perinatal deaths.

Inadequate nutrition and poor maternal education have been linked to the unacceptably high stillbirth and neonatal deaths in low income countries. Poorly fed mothers either early in childhood or later in life may lead to low birthweight which is one of the significant contributors to perinatal mortality. Poor maternal education is not only associated with poor nutrition but poor health seeking behaviour and poor perinatal outcome.

Certain maternal health conditions such as pregnancy-induced or essential hypertension, diabetes mellitus, anaemia and infections (Malaria, HIV and tuberculosis) predispose to intrauterine growth retardation (IUGR), low birth weight and perinatal death. Poor birth spacing with inter birth interval of less than 2 years leading to poor maternal nutritional reserves predisposes women to low birth weight infants and perinatal death. Maternal status of high parity and extremes of age (less than 18 years and greater than 45 years) are associated with poor birth outcomes and perinatal morbidity and mortality. Low socioeconomic status of the mother has been shown to be associated with higher perinatal mortality rate.

Effective and appropriate maternal interventions such as micronutrient supplementation, intermittent presumptive treatment (IPTp) of malaria and tetanus toxoid vaccination cannot be offered if women do not avail themselves of antenatal services. Several studies in low income countries has shown that a large proportion of perinatal deaths occur in women who did not receive antenatal care during pregnancy [15].

Poorly supervised labour either in a hospital setting or conducted outside a health facility by persons ill equipped to manage labour and delivery is a major cause of stillbirth and early neonatal death. Unskilled attendance at delivery and inadequate resuscitation of the newborn predispose to birth asphyxia and death. Unsanitary conditions when deliveries are conducted in inappropriate places pave the way for early neonatal sepsis and eventual death.

Prenatal complications such as antepartum haemorrhage secondary to placenta praevia or abruptio placenta; pre eclampsia or eclampsia all predispose to fetal loss. In addition complications during labour and delivery such as cord prolapse and uterine rupture may lead to still births or birth asphyxia.

Multiple pregnancies are associated withpreterm delivery and low birth weight which are leading causes of perinatal morbidity and mortality.

The real causes of adverse fetal and early neonatal outcomes in the low income countries of sub Saharan Africa and South central Asia are inadequate obstetric and neonatal care, and harmful home care practices, such as the discarding of colostrum, the application of unclean substances to the umbilical cord stump, and the failure to keep babies warm [3].

5. Strategies to reduce perinatal mortality

In many parts of the world up to half of deliveries still take place at home without adequate supervision. This is even higher in the developing countries especially of sub-Saharan Africa and could be due to cultural practices that stipulate that certain births must take place in the home. Poor access to health facilities as a result of unavailability or financial constraints; lack of faith in health systems because of inadequate facility, manpower or poor attitude of health care workers, or just plain ignorance of the benefits of skilled attendance at deliveries all contribute to adverse prenatal outcome[,15,16 17]. Also in some deeply religious settings such as are found in many African countries, a significant proportion of births occur in spiritual/mission homes with unskilled or poorly skilled attendants. All these practice predispose to perinatal mortality [15,16,17] .

Reducing perinatal mortality is a prerequisite for attaining MDG 4. Increased investment in health by various governments is necessary to tackle the factors predisposing to the unacceptably high perinatal mortality rates in low income countries. Strengthening of Health Systems includes provision of sufficient number of well-equipped health facilities and with proportional spread to meet local needs. Health facilities for the management of uncomplicated pregnancies and deliveries should be within the reach of every woman in every community. The peripheral centres should be linked to centrally-located secondary level health facilities with capacity for assisted or operative deliveries and some advanced care for the newborns. Regional tertiary centres with facilities to manage high risk pregnancies and deliveries as well as special care baby units with facilities for neonatal intensive care should also be established. There should be well established 2-way referral system between one level of health facility and the next.

In most low income countries like Nigeria, though these three levels of care exist, appropriate referral linkages from one level of healthcare to the next are lacking making the health system inefficient and dysfunctional [16,17] .The roads linking these facilities, as well as appropriate transport systems are in terrible disrepair or non-existent. In most low income countries, most deliveries are supervised by unskilled birth attendants. Efforts over the years have been devoted to training these unskilled attendants with no appreciable success [17]. If the MDG 4 must be achieved by 2015, investment should be directed at training a critical mass of health workers with sufficient basic education to understand the science and techniques of perinatology. The capacity of health workers in this setting with high perinatal mortality should be strengthened to meet the needs of women during pregnancy and delivery as well as provide appropriate care for newborns. All doctors, nurses and midwives should be trained on basic neonatal resuscitation. In low income countries were traditional birth attendants supervise a large proportion of deliveries they should be retrained as community liaisons officers- with the responsibility to link the women and their families to health facility. Specialist skills in obstetrics and neonatology need to be built among healthcare workers to care for high risk pregnancies, deliveries and newborns. Specialist skills acquisition is particularly urgent in the low income countries to man the regional referral centres. Mal-distribution of the specialized care needs to be addressed in some countries like Nigeria where there is concentration of highly skilled staff and health care workers in city centres where less than 20% of the population resides.

Access to maternal and child health facilities should be improved by either the removal of user fees at these facilities or by introducing affordable and accessible community based health insurance schemes that ensure that the poorest of the poor have access to these facilities.

Women empowerment through education of the girl child and the introduction of poverty alleviation programmes are long term strategies that though may not have immediate impact on perinatal mortality are essential for sustaining the rate once achieved with some quick win interventions.

Finally abolition of harmful cultural practices detrimental to fetal and neonatal survival and early detection and treatment of malformations and genetic diseases will all in no mean measure contribute to reduction in perinatal mortality.

6. Conclusion

Low income countries account for 97-98 percent of reported global perinatal deaths. This accounts for 68-70% of annual global under five mortality. It is therefore not possible to achieve the stated MDG 4 goal of reducing infant mortality rate by two thirds of 1990 rates by 2015 without addressing the causes and determinants of perinatal mortality especially in these low income countries. Many useful interventions can be implemented in resource-poor settings, but weak health care delivery systems remain a major challenge.

Urgently required are alternative approaches to deploy the evidence proven strategies that had led to the reduction of perinatal mortality in high and medium income countries.

7. References

[1] WHO. The world health report 2005: make every mother and child count. Geneva: World Health Organization, 2005.

[2] WHO. Neonatal and perinatal mortality: Country, Regional and Global Estimates. World Health Organization 2006

[3] Zupan J, Aahman E. Perinatal mortality for the year 2000: estimates developed by WHO. Geneva: World Health Organization, 2005

[4] Zupan J. Perinatal Mortality in Developing Countries. N. Engl J Med 2005; 352(20):2047-2048

[5] UNICEF. Levels and trends in child mortality report . UNICEF 2010

[6] Lawn JE, Cousens S, Zupan. 4 million neonatal deaths: When? Where? Why? Lancet 2005; 365: 891–900

[7] Richardus JH, Graafmans WC, Verloove-Vanhorick SP, Mackenbach JP. The perinatal mortality rate as an indicator of quality of care in international comparisons. Med Care. 1998; 36 (1):54.

[8] Cousens S, Stanton C, Blencowe H, et al. National, regional, and worldwide estimates of stillbirth rates in 2009 with trends since1995: a systematic analysis. *Lancet* 2011; published online April 14.DOI:10.1016/S0140-6736 (10)62310-0.

[9] Rajaratnam JK, Marcus JR, Flaxman AD, Wang H, Levin-Recto A, Dwyer Let al. Neonatal, post neonatal, childhood, and under-5 mortality for 187 countries, 1970–2010: a systematic analysis of progress towards Millennium Development Goal 4. Lancet 2010; 375: 1988–2008.

[10] Akpala CO. Perinatal mortality in a northern Nigerian rural community. *J R Soc Health* 1993; 113: 124–27.

[11] Aisien AO, Lawson JO, Okolo A. Two years prospective study of perinatal mortality in Jos, Nigeria. *Int J Gynaecol Obstet* 2000; 71: 171-73.

[12] MacDorman MF, Kirmeyer S. Fetal and perinatal mortality, United States, 2005. *Natl Vital Stat Rep* 2009; 57: 1–19

[13] Flenady V, Koopmans L, Middleton P, et al. Major risk factors for stillbirth in high-income countries: a systematic review and meta-analysis. *Lancet* 2011; published online April 14. DOI:10.1016/S0140-6736(10)62233-7.

[14] Black ER, Cousens S, Johnson HL, Lawn JE, Rudan I, Bassani DG et al. Global, regional, and national causes of child mortality in 2008: a systematic analysis. Lancet 2010; 375: 1969–87

[15] Ezechi OC, Fasubaa OB, Dare FO: Socioeconomic barrier to safe motherhood among booked patients in rural Nigerian communities. Journal of Obstetrics and Gynaecology 2000, 20(1):32-34.

[16] Idris SH, Gwarzo UMD, Shehu AU. Determinants of place of delivery among women in a semi-urban settlement in Zaria, Northern Nigeria. Annals of African Medicine. 2006;5(1):68-72

[17] Ezechi OC, Fasuba OB, Obiesie OB, Kalu BKE, Loto OM, Ndububa VI, Olomola O. Delivery outside hospital after antenatal care: prevalence and its predictors. 2004; 24(7);745-749

2

The Effect of Intrauterine Development and Nutritional Status on Perinatal, Intrauterine and Neonatal Mortality: The MDN System

Péter Berkő[1] and Kálmán Joubert[2]
[1]*Faculty of Healthcare, Miskolc University, Department of Obstetrics and Gynaecology, Borsod-Abaúj-Zemplén County and University Teaching Hospital, Miskolc*
[2]*Demographic Research Institute, Central Statistic Office, Budapest*
Hungary

1. Introduction

Obstetricians and neonatologists have since long made efforts to estimate precisely the life chances of neonates soon after their birth, even in the delivery room. The objective is twofold: to diagnose possible diseases and recognise and differentiate the neonates who are highly endangered because of the deficiencies and disorders of their bodily development.

The most common method is still in use: by measuring the bodyweights of neonates, one can immediately differentiate those whose weights are below 2,500 grams, and who are regarded as being the most endangered newborns. Recently, however, specialists normally differentiate between neonates of body weight below 1,500 grams, those less than 1,000 grams and those who weigh less than 500 grams at birth. At the same time, we have learned that body weight alone is not a reliable parameter to estimate the life chances of a neonate (Macferlene et al., 1980, WHO, 1961, 1970, Wilcox & Russel, 1983, 1990). This is true for a series of reasons: (1) body weight depends on many factors; (2) each weight group is extremely heterogeneous when gestational age, body length and nutritional status (nourishment) are considered (Berkő, 1992, Berkő & Joubert, 2006, 2009, Zadik et al., 2003), however, scientific research needs homogeneous groups to study; (3) since the average birth weights of neonate populations differ greatly by country and race (Meredith, 1970), there is no practical chance to develop uniform weight criteria to be applicable in each country.

Another option is to determine the gestational ages of neonates in order to differentiate highly endangered or preterm babies. As the survival chance correlates with gestational age rather than with birthweight, in 1961 WHO declared that not a birth weight below 2500 grams, but neonates born before the 37th week have to be considered as premature (WHO, 1961).

Lubchenco was the first to recognise that body weight and gestational age have to be considered simultaneously in order to determine the bodily development of a neonate (Lubchenco et al., 1963). On the basis of the birth standards developed by Battaglia & Lubchenco (1967), it was recommended that newborns below the 10th weight percentile, or

SGA (small for gestational age), were qualified as being highly endangered. Later on, SGA neonates were referred to as having intrauterine growth retardation (IUGR), because many newborns in the weight group under the 10th weight percentile were found to have retardation syndrome.

However, it was revealed later that the clinical picture of retardation is not a uniform syndrome, taking into account its etiology, clinical picture and prognosis (Bakketeig, 1998, Battaglia and Lubchenco, 1967, Deorari et al., 2001, Doszpod, 2000, Golde, 1989, Gruenwald, 1963, 1966, Henriksen, 1999, Kurjak et al., 1978, Kramer et al., 1990, Lin et al., 1991, Lin, 1998, Rosso & Winick, 1974, Senterre, 1989, Wollmann, 1998). As a basic requirement, one has to be able to differentiate between proportionally and disproportionally retarded newborn babies. One can only do that if gestational age and birth weight body length is also considered (Abernathy et al., 1996, Golde, 1989, Kramer et al., 1990, Miller & Hassanein, 1971). Rohrer's Ponderal Index (Hassanein, 1971, Rohrer, 1961) was introduced for this purpose, but it was not commonly used, because the database to calculate the index was limited and the proposed mathematical formula [(gram/cm^3)x100] was not popular. Nevertheless, more and more authors underline the need for the consideration of nutritional status.

Recent scientific results confirm the recognition that the development and nutritional statuses of foetuses and neonates have a major impact on their viability, their intrauterineand neonatal morbidity (Kadi and Gardosi, 2004, Shrimpton, 2003), as well as on their morbidity in adulthood (Barker et al., 1993, Goldfrey & Barker, 2000, Gyenis et al., 2004, Henriksen, 1999, Joubert & Gyenis, 2003, Osmond & Barker, 2000). It also has been proven that development and nutritional status at birth influence the growth rate, bodily development, and the intellectual faculties of a child up until 18 years of age (Joubert & Gyenis, 2003).

The authors firmly believe that more accurate estimations of the survival chances and the degree of endangeredness of neonates can be achieved if the three important factors are simultaneously considered: (i) maturity (gestational age); (ii) bodily development (weight and length standard positions determined on the basis of appropriate weight and length standards); (iii) nutritional status depending upon the relative weight and length development. However, the question is how to consider all of these factors at the same time, and more importantly, how to differentiate less endangered and highly endangered neonate groups identified in this complex system of classification. The authors developed a new method to achieve this.

In the present study the authors describe their novel method, the MDN system (MDN: Maturity, Development, Nutritional status) (Berkő, 1992, Berkő & Joubert, 2006, 2009) and its application:

- to determine the nutritional status of a neonate on the basis of its gestational age, length and weight delopment considered simultaneously;
- to differentiate the most viable and the most endangered neonates on the basis of their development and nutritional status;
- to demonstrate the influence of a neonate's bodily development and nutritional status by intrauterine, neonatal and perinatal mortality rate.

- to identify and distinguish those retarded neonates who are likely to need growth hormone treatment in the future.

2. Method – The MDN system

The MDN system, integrating four important birth parameters, offers a method to decide to what extent a neonate is endangered on the basis of its bodily development and nutritional status. The four parameters: sex, gestational age, birth weight and birth length.

2.1 The determination of weight and length standard positions

The weight and length development of a newborn is determined on the basis of its sex, gestational age, body mass and length at birth. To do this, however, sex-specific national weight and length standards of reference value are needed. In Hungary, Joubert prepared such standards on the basis of the birth data of babies born in this country between 1990 and 1996 (799,688 neonates) (Joubert, 2000). As is the case with other commonly known standards, Joubert's standards apply 7 percentile curves (percentiles 3, 10, 25, 50, 75, 90 and 97) to divide the entire weight and length ranges into 8 weight zones and 8 length zones. The field under percentile curve 3 forms zone 1; zone 2 is made by the area between percentile curves 3 and 10, while the area above percentile curve 97 gives zone 8 (as shown in Tables 1-4).

Zones	Percen-tiles	Gestational weeks																								Percen-tiles
		20	21	22	23	24	25	26	27	28	29	30	31	32	33	34	35	36	37	38	39	40	41	42	43	
8																										
	97	705	775	845	925	1019	1129	1269	1425	1615	1825	2055	2285	2545	2787	3048	3325	3579	3819	4018	4193	4349	4495	4595	4627	97
7																										
	90	595	665	735	815	895	995	1119	1259	1435	1616	1828	2055	2277	2508	2755	3008	3276	3525	3729	3909	4075	4195	4295	4328	90
6																										
	75	525	585	645	718	795	888	995	1128	1295	1475	1649	1845	2048	2259	2488	2725	2976	3238	3458	3655	3795	3895	3955	3979	75
5																										
	50	455	501	555	621	705	781	881	1005	1155	1311	1481	1659	1851	2045	2255	2475	2721	2949	3161	3349	3495	3608	3655	3671	50
4																										
	25	385	422	475	533	595	685	782	895	1015	1152	1305	1455	1615	1805	2005	2211	2425	2663	2875	3055	3213	3305	3341	3352	25
3																										
	10	311	351	395	455	515	595	683	775	881	995	1123	1253	1395	1561	1745	1935	2164	2395	2623	2805	2925	3005	3035	3021	10
2																										
	3	245	275	315	361	422	482	561	643	725	833	935	1051	1182	1323	1493	1671	1872	2105	2322	2524	2672	2754	2762	2735	3
1																										

Table 1. Weight standards for the Hungarian male neonates born between 1990 and 1996 (grames)

Zones	Percen-tiles	Gestational weeks																								Percen-tiles
		20	21	22	23	24	25	26	27	28	29	30	31	32	33	34	35	36	37	38	39	40	41	42	43	
8																										
	97	36.9	39.1	41.1	42.9	44.6	46.2	47.6	49.1	50.5	51.6	52.7	53.6	54.5	55.3	56.2	56.9	57.5	58.1	58.5	58.8	59.1	59.2	59.3	59.4	97
7																										
	90	34.1	36.2	38.3	40.2	41.9	43.5	44.9	46.5	47.8	49.1	50.3	51.3	52.3	53.3	54.2	54.9	55.7	56.4	56.9	57.4	57.6	57.8	57.9	57.9	90
6																										
	75	31.8	33.9	35.8	37.7	39.4	40.9	42.5	43.9	45.3	46.6	47.9	49.1	50.2	51.3	52.3	53.1	53.8	54.5	55.1	55.4	55.6	55.8	55.9	55.9	75
5																										
	50	29.5	31.4	33.3	35.1	36.9	38.6	40.1	41.6	42.9	44.3	45.7	46.9	48.1	49.3	50.4	51.3	52.1	52.7	53.2	53.5	53.7	53.9	53.9	54.1	50
4																										
	25	27.1	29.1	30.8	32.7	34.3	36.1	37.6	39.1	40.7	42.1	43.5	44.7	46.1	47.2	48.4	49.5	50.3	50.9	51.4	51.8	52.1	52.2	52.2	52.3	25
3																										
	10	24.4	26.5	28.3	30.2	31.9	33.5	35.1	36.7	38.3	39.9	41.3	42.7	44.1	45.4	46.5	47.8	48.6	49.3	49.9	50.2	50.4	50.4	50.5	50.5	10
2																										
	3	21.6	23.4	25.2	27.2	28.9	30.7	32.3	33.9	35.4	36.9	38.5	40.1	41.8	43.2	44.8	46.1	47.1	47.8	48.2	48.6	48.8	48.9	48.9	49.1	3
1																										

Table 2. Length standards for the Hungarian male neonates born between 1990 and 1996 (centimetres)

Zones	Percentiles	Gestational weeks 20	21	22	23	24	25	26	27	28	29	30	31	32	33	34	35	36	37	38	39	40	41	42	43	Percentiles
8																										
	97	675	725	801	895	995	1118	1269	1438	1638	1845	2055	2295	2545	2775	3015	3239	3466	3669	3855	4025	4176	4315	4368	4355	**97**
7																										
	90	595	635	689	765	849	965	1096	1245	1417	1605	1796	2005	2235	2455	2685	2917	3155	3375	3568	3747	3898	4005	4055	4049	**90**
6																										
	75	529	555	601	668	755	855	968	1097	1255	1425	1615	1805	2018	2225	2438	2655	2885	3098	3296	3475	3619	3725	3775	3798	**75**
5																										
	50	461	479	521	582	655	749	852	967	1101	1255	1425	1602	1803	1998	2201	2402	2617	2835	3035	3202	3329	3415	3475	3497	**50**
4																										
	25	395	415	451	501	573	651	751	855	975	1105	1245	1402	1581	1765	1952	2145	2355	2565	2773	2945	3075	3161	3202	3205	**25**
3																										
	10	335	352	382	425	481	562	643	735	843	953	1072	1201	1355	1525	1701	1891	2103	2325	2525	2703	2835	2912	2943	2951	**10**
2																										
	3	282	295	323	355	405	465	531	614	702	791	885	1003	1132	1283	1455	1645	1845	2052	2255	2455	2614	2701	2725	2732	**3**
1																										

Table 3. Weight standards for the Hungarian female neonates born between 1990 and 1996 (grames)

Zones	Percentiles	Gestational weeks 20	21	22	23	24	25	26	27	28	29	30	31	32	33	34	35	36	37	38	39	40	41	42	43	Percentiles
8																										
	97	37.5	39.3	41.3	43.1	44.8	46.4	47.9	49.3	50.5	51.7	52.7	53.5	54.5	55.2	55.9	56.5	57.1	57.5	57.8	58.1	58.3	58.4	58.5	58.6	**97**
7																										
	90	34.8	36.5	38.5	40.2	41.8	43.5	45.2	46.7	48.1	49.2	50.3	51.3	52.2	53.1	53.7	54.4	55.1	55.6	56.1	56.4	56.6	56.8	56.9	56.9	**90**
6																										
	75	32.1	33.9	35.6	37.3	39.1	40.8	42.5	43.9	45.4	46.8	47.9	49.1	50.1	51.1	51.9	52.7	53.3	53.9	54.4	54.7	54.9	55.2	55.3	55.4	**75**
5																										
	50	28.8	30.8	32.9	34.7	36.5	38.1	39.6	41.1	42.6	43.9	45.3	46.5	47.7	48.7	49.7	50.5	51.3	51.9	52.4	52.9	53.2	53.4	53.5	53.5	**50**
4																										
	25	26.1	28.1	30.1	32.1	33.9	35.8	37.5	39.1	40.4	41.9	43.2	44.4	45.7	46.9	47.9	48.9	49.7	50.3	50.8	51.1	51.3	51.5	51.6	51.6	**25**
3																										
	10	23.1	25.3	27.2	29.3	31.3	33.1	34.9	36.6	38.1	39.6	41.1	42.4	43.8	44.9	46.2	47.2	47.9	48.5	49.1	49.4	49.6	49.8	49.9	49.9	**10**
2																										
	3	20.1	22.1	24.1	26.1	28.1	30.1	31.9	33.7	35.3	36.8	38.3	39.8	41.2	42.6	43.9	45.2	46.2	46.8	47.4	47.7	47.9	48.1	48.2	48.3	**3**
1																										

Table 4. Length standards for Hungarian female neonates born between 1990 and 1996 (centimetres)

By using tabulated standards or software designed specifically for the purpose, knowing the gestational age one can easily determine the weight zone (W) and length zone (L) of a newborn baby on the basis of its weight and length at birth. Any neonate can be described with the letters (W and L) and numbers (1-8) of its weight and length zones. For example, if the birth weight of a newborn is in weight zone 6, i.e., between weight percentile curves 75 and 90, and its length is in length zone 2, i.e., between percentile curves 3 and 10, then the standard positions of this baby are W6 and L2.

2.2 Description of the nutritional status

To characterize and decribe the nutritional status of the newborn (N) one should know the relation of his weight standard position (W) to his own length standard position (L). The authors prepared a matrix comprising eight horizontal lines for the weight standard zones and eight columns for the length standard zones, which seems a useful tool to determine the nutritional status of neonates. This 64-cell matrix is referred to as the MDN matrix (see Figure 1, where the neonate mentioned earlier as [W6, L2] is positioned in the grey cell). Any newborn can be positioned in this table, no matter what weight or length zone it belongs to. Each cell is identified by the letter and number of the weight zone and of the length zone, in the intersection of which the cell is located in the matrix.

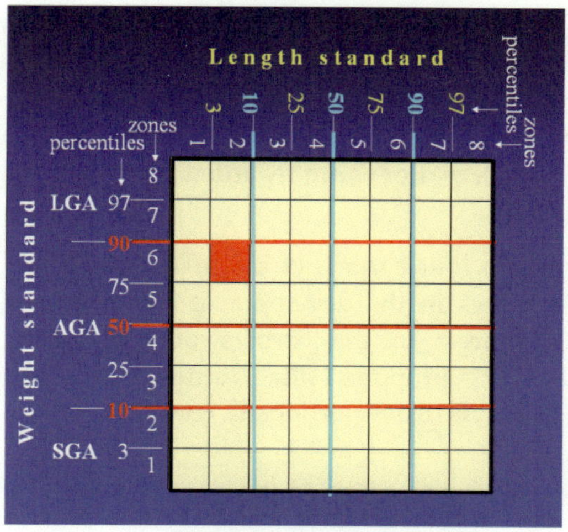

Fig. 1. MDN matrix for the simultaneous representation of weight and length standard positions of neonates. Neonates in cell W6-L2 belong to weight standard zone 6 (between percentile curves 90 and 97) and to length standard zone 2 (between percentile curves 3 and 10).

In order to describe nutritional status (N) of a neonate, one has to know its weight standard position (weight zone number = W) and length standard position (length zone number = L). The calculation of the nutritional index, or nourishment status: N = W – L. If the number of the weight zone is higher than that of the length zone, then N will be a positive number, which means that the baby is born with a relative overweight (overnourished). When N is a negative number, the baby is relatively underweight for its length. Using the example above, (W6,L2) works out to N=+4, or an overnourished baby.

Figure 2 demonstrates the nutritional status (N value) of neonates in each cell of the 64-cell MDN matrix. The N value, representing nutritional status as rated according to the

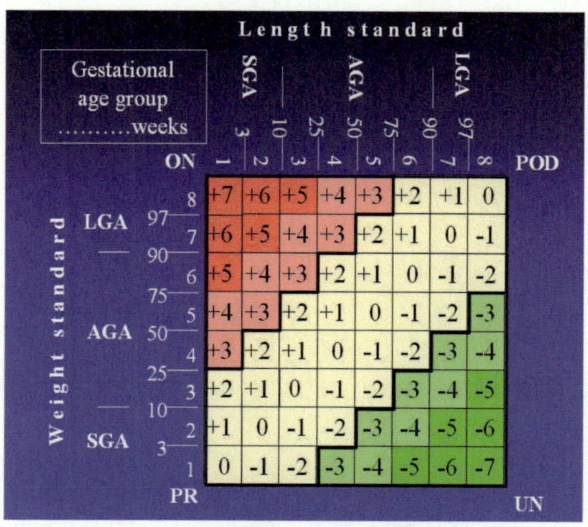

Fig. 2. The weight and length standard positions (W and L) and N values (W-L) of neonates with different nutritional statuses in the MDN matrix. The corners of the MDN matrix: PR (proportionally retarded), POD (proportionally overdeveloped), ON (overnourished), UN (undernourished).

matrix, can range from +7 to -7. Obviously, extremely overnourished neonates are positioned in the cells marked +5,+6,+7, while extremely undernourished ones will be positioned in the cells marked -5,-6,-7. In an ideal case, a neonate is positioned in the weight zone and length zone having identical numbers when its N value = 0. Neonates with N = 0, N = +1 or +2 and those with N = -1 or -2 are regarded as being normally (or proportionally) nourished.

For better understanding, the four corners of the MDN matrix are marked with letters to indicate the typical differences in the development and nutritional statuses of neonates positioned in the cells nearest to the corners of the matrix. Abbreviations: PR = proportionally retarded, POD = proportionally overdeveloped, ON = overnourished, UN = under-nourished (or DPR, that is disproportionally retarded).

2.3 Classification of neonates according to the degree of nourishment

On an MDN matrix the gestational age-group should always indicate the appropriate data from the standards tables. Figure 3 and Table 5 demonstrate the most typical groups of newborns according to their nourishment. The figure also demonstrates the incidence rates of neonates with specific development and nutritional status in the neonate population born in Hungary between 1997 and 2003 (680,947 newborn babies as recorded by the Hungarian Statistical Office). About 90.6% of the Hungarian newborns are averagely nourished. Of these, 25.8% were at an "absolutely normal" level of development and nourishment. The incidence of the undernourished group (UN, which we consider to be disproportionally retarded) is 4.5%. The ratio of overnourishment (ON) is 4.9%. The percentage of proportionally retarded (PR) neonates who are likely to need growth hormone therapy is 4.5%. In the Figure 3, below the 10th percentile – in the weight zone W1-2 - a mixed group of retarded is to be found among the proportionally and disproportionally retarded neonates (Berkő, 1996). Looking at the figure it is easy to recognize that the so-called SGA-born infants form a highly heterogeneous group. This fact implies that it is wrong to consider the SGA group as a whole to be the potential ones to receive growth hormone treatment, since

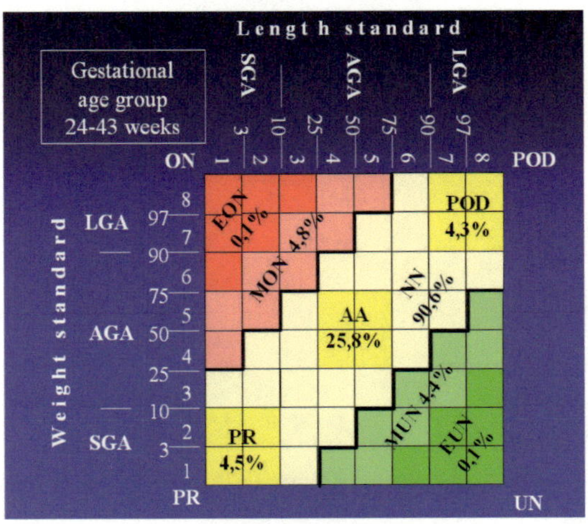

Fig. 3. The classification (and percentage distribution) of Hungarian neonates born between 1997 and 2003 by bodily development and nourishment.

only growth of the proportionally retarded or possibly the mixed group of retarded neonates (MR) will lag behind the average.

Table 5 shows how to define and separate the most characteristic groups of neonates according to their differing nutritional status.

Nourishment	Abbreviations	Position on the MDN table	Prevalence %
Overnourished	ON	N = +3 - +7	4.9
extremely overnourished	EON	N = +5, +6, +7	0.1
moderately overnourished	MON	N = +3, +4	4.8
Normally nourished	NN	N = -2 - +2	90.6
proportionally overdeveloped	POD	W7-8, L7-8	4.3
absolute average	AA	W 4-5 L4-5	25.8
proportionally retarded	PR	W1-2 L1-2	4.5
Undernourished (disproportionally retarded, DPR)	UN (DPR)	N = -3 - -7	4.5
moderately undernourished	MUN	N = -3, -4	4.4
extremely undernourished	EUN	N = -5, -6, -7	0.1

Table 5. Most typical groups of newborns according to their nourishment

2.4 The numerical representation of neonates by their maturity, weight and length with the help of the MDN index

As explained earlier, the MDN method is a tool to describe the maturity, bodily development and nutritional status of any neonate numerically. The *MDN index = GA / W / L / N,* where GA is gestational age in weeks; W is a number that demonstrates which zone the numeric weight score belongs to (1 to 8); L is the corresponding score of the body-length standard (1 to 8); N=W-L, the score of the nutritional status. If N is a positive number, this means that the baby is born with a relative overweight (overnourished, ON). When N is a negative number, the baby is relatively underweight for its length. The group of UN neonates can be characterized as disproportionally retarded (DPR)._Examples: (a) MDN index is GA=38 / W= 6 / L= 2 / N= +4; (b) MDN index is GA=38 / W= 2 / L= 6 / N= -4 (Berkő and Joubert, 2006, 2009).

3. The effect of bodily development and nutritional status on perinatal mortality

By processing the birth data of the entire neonate population, gestational age 24-43 weeks, born in Hungary in the years 1997 to 2003, the authors studied the perinatal mortality rate of the neonates in each cell of the MDN matrix (Figure 4). The four cells in the centre of the table represent the neonates considered an *absolute average* (AA) or etalon group on the basis of their weight and length.

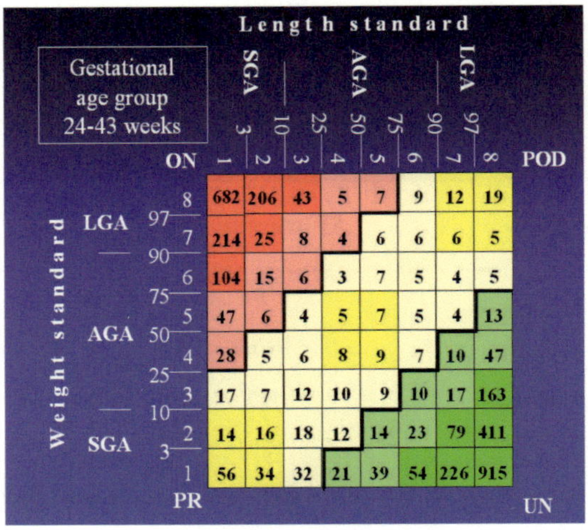

Fig. 4. Perinatal mortality rates (‰) of the entire Hungarian neonate population (gestational age 24-43 weeks) born between 1997 and 2003, as represented by the cells of the MDN matrix.

Relying on the birth data of neonates born between 1997 and 2003, the authors find *perinatal mortality rate to be 8.9‰*in Hungary in that period of time. For comparison, this rate in the absolute average group, which is necessary to determine for comparative studies, was 7‰ in the same period of time. The highlighted sectors of the MDN matrix in Figure 5 represent the most endangered neonate groups.

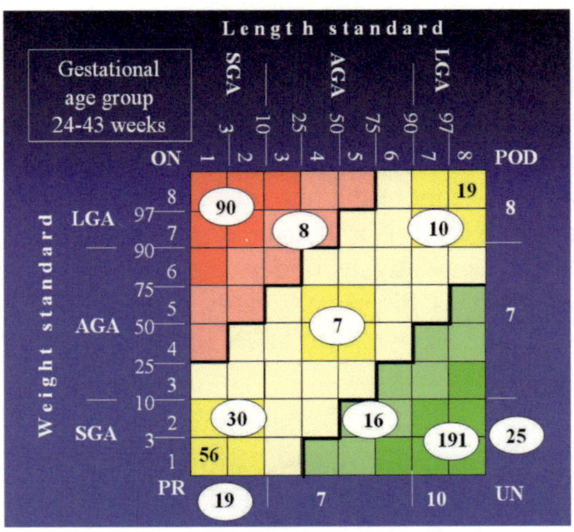

Fig. 5. Perinatal mortality rates (‰) in the major groups of the Hungarian neonate population (gestational age 24-43 weeks) born between 1997 and 2003, which are regarded as being the most endangered groups on the basis of bodily development and nutritional status (as represented in the major sectors of the MDN table)

3.1 The major groups of highly endangered foetuses and neonates with the help of the MDN matrix

Undernourished (UN) group. These babies were born with insufficient weight and often show the syndrome of classic **disproportional retardation.** The perinatal mortality rate is rather high, 21‰ in the large group of undernourished neonates. The group comprises the moderately undernourished subgroup with a PM rate of merely 16‰. The cells creating the triangle of extremely undernourished neonates (EUN) in the UN corner of the table have a conspicuously high PM rate of 191‰. The MDN table clearly shows that disproportional retardation, which causes a high mortality rate, can be found not only among the neonates under weight percentile 10, but also among those over weight percentile 10, as two-thirds of the investigated cases show.

Overnourished (ON) group. The PM rate is 10‰ in the overnourished group. This group includes the moderately overnourished subgroup where the PM rate is only 8‰. The PM rate is 90‰ in the triangle of the extremely overnourished group (EON) in the ON corner of the MDN Table.

Proportionally retarded (PR) group. Proportionally retarded babies are positioned in the four bottom left cells (in the PR corner) giving the field bordered by weight percentile 10 and length percentile 10. The PM rate in this group is 30‰. However, the smallest disproportionally retarded neonates, being under percentile 3 by both weight and length (EPR), have an even higher PM rate of 56‰.

Proportionally overdeveloped group. The group of extremely proportionally overdeveloped (EOD) or giant babies should not be overlooked. They are positioned in the POD corner of the table, with both their weight and length in the 8th percentile zone. They are also highly endangered, as is shown by the 19‰ PM rate of this cell.

Perinatal mortality in the heterogeneous SGA group. PM rate in the weight group under the 10th percentile (heterogeneous SGA by length and nutritional status) is 25‰ (in the AGA group it is 7‰, and 8‰ in the LGA group, which is over the 90th percentile). A very high PM rate of 43‰ is found in the weight group under the 3rd percentile.

3.2 The effect of bodily development and nutritional status on perinatal mortality in the groups of Hungarian premature and mature infants

By comparing the perinatal mortality (PM) of Hungarian preterm and full-term neonates, using the data given in Figure 6, we can conclude the following: (1) absolutely averagely developed and nourished (AA) preterm infant mortality is 28 times as high as that of the full-term AA group, and (2) independently of gestational age disproportional retardation (DPR), extreme overnourishment (EON) and proportional retardation (PR) significantly enhance the perinatal mortality risk of preterms born in the 24th-36th gestational week compared to that of full-term neonates (37th-42nd gestational week).

4. Criticism of the "perinatal mortality" indicator

Perinatal mortality (PM) is one of the most important parameters of public health indicator data. It describes the incidence of late (24 weeks or older) fetal intrauterine death, plus the perinatal (1st to 7th day) death incidence of the live-born fetuses of the population studied. In standard practice, this is the only indicator with which we can draw conclusions on prenatal care, delivery room care and neonatal care quality level. I believe that now is the time for us to realize that the PM is not really suitable for this purpose (Berkő, 2006). Why?

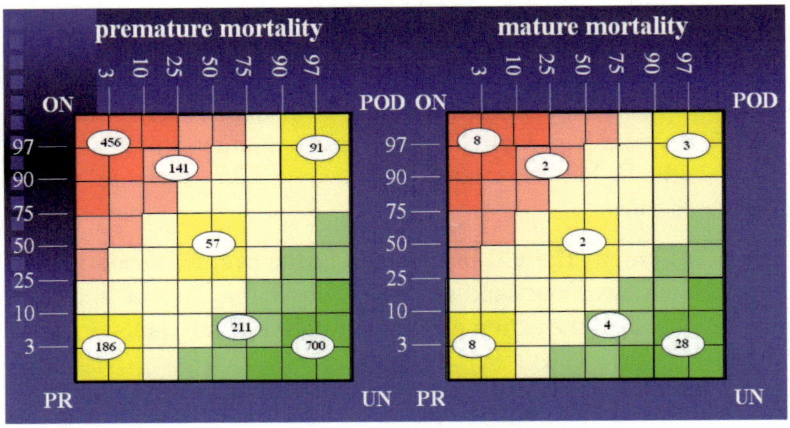

Fig. 6. Comparison of perinatal mortality of the premature and mature Hungarian infants with the help of the MDN matrix.

4.1 Intrauterine and neonatal mortality rate is also important to know

Morbidity and mortality parameters are useful when they also reveal the cause of the particular disease or death. PM is not suitable for this. In Hungary, perinatal mortality in 2007 (in two counties) was 11.1‰. But while in one of the three counties, County A, the intrauterine fetal mortality incidence was 3.6‰ and the neonate mortality 7.5‰, County B's situation was vice-versa, with intrauterine death at 7.3‰ and a perinatal (1st to 7th day of life) mortality rate of 3.8‰. It is quite obvious that there are problems with neonatal care in County A, while County B suffers from inappropriate prenatal care. If we only possess the average information of 11.1‰ perinatal mortality for both counties, there is no mode for recognition of such problems, nor is there any opportunity to set tasks for specific care improvement. Therefore I propose that each case of perinatal mortality rate should be supplemented with the two components of the PM: intrauterine and perinatal mortality.

4.2 Extention of the "perinatal period" concept should be considered!

But there is another problem. The concept of PM along with intrauterine death includes also mortality occurring on Day 1-7 postpartum. This is unacceptable nowadays. Hungary clearly shows that there is no reason for feeling satisfied, since along with declining perinatal mortality (1st-7th day after delivery) a continuous parallel increase of 8th-28th day neonatal mortality has been observed. The explanation for this is that the use of modern medications and breathing support allows us to extend the life of many small prematurely born infants, whom we lose only after the 7th day of their lives. With this in mind, therefore, I propose to introduce the concept of "*extended perinatal mortality*" *(EPM)*, which includes intrauterine deaths (IUM) and live-born infant Day 1-28 mortality (NM).

In view of facts described above, let us graphically represent the perinatal (PM), intrauterine (IU) and neonatal (NM, day 1-28) Hungarian mortality data of 1997-2003 in correlation with bodily development and nutritional status (Figure 7 and Table 6). It is clear to see that growth retardation and overnourishment nearly identically increase the intrauterine and

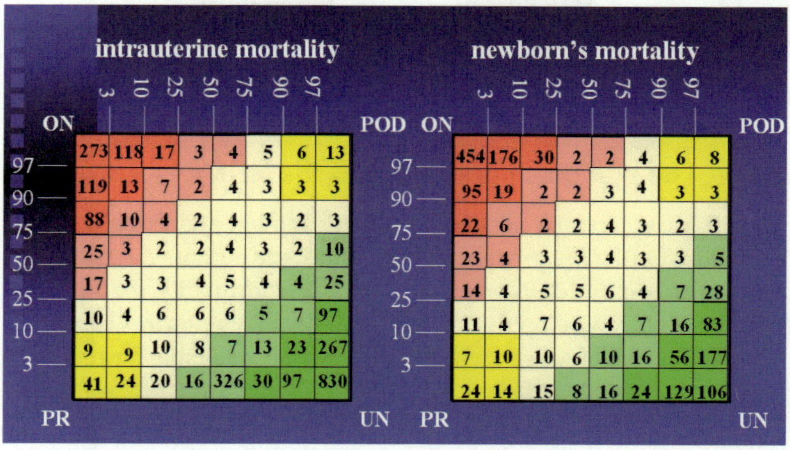

Fig. 7. Comparison of intrauterine and neonate mortality (‰) based on the MDN matrix

Nourishment	Abbre-viations	Perinatal mortality (‰)	Intrauterine mortality (‰)	Day 1-28 neonatal mortality (‰)	Extended perinatal mortality (‰)
680,947 newborns, 1997-2003		8.9	4.3	5.1	9.4
Overnourished	ON	10	6	5	11
extremely ON	EON	90	51	49	100
moderately ON	MON	8	5	5	10
Normally nourished	NN	9	5	5	10
proportionally overdeveloped	POD	10	6	5	11
absolute average	AA	7	4	4	8
proportionally retarded	PR	30	20	14	34
Undernourished (disproportionally retarded)	UN (DPR)	21	12	12	24
moderately UN	MUN	16	9	10	19
extremely UN	EUN	191	124	78	202
Weight for gestational age					
large	LGA	8	5	8	13
average	AGA	7	4	7	11
small	SGA	25	17	25	42

Table 6. Intrauterine and perinatal (1-28 day) mortality according to the most characteristic development and nutritional groups of newborns

neonatal mortality rate. Is also obvious that following groups are most at risk, in descending order: in greatest danger - the group of extremely undernourished (severe disproportional retardation) (EUN), extremely overnourished (EON), and proportionally retarded (PR), followed by the group of extremely proportionally retarded (EPR). A significantly higher mortality rate can also be observed among the proportionally overdeveloped neonates (POD, respectively EPOD). Figure 7 proves that a significant deviation in physical development and nourishment from the average (i.e., the PR, EON, DPR groups) is of great danger to both foetuses in utero and and neonates (Day 1-28).

5. Conclusion – The practical importance of the MDN system

Relying on the empirical fact that the degree of nourishment and the status of development have a high influence on the life prospects of neonates, the authors developed a method, the MDN system - including an MDN matrix - to study and qualify the nutritional status at birth. The MDN system can be applied when gestational age, birth weight and length are known and when reliable weight and length standards are available for reference.

The MDN index provides an easy and short numerical characterization of every newborn according to its state of maturity, bodily development and nutritional status. This requires only four parameters : MDN index = GA / W / L / N (gestational age, weight, length, nutritional status).

The MDN matrix enables effective separation into groups according to their mortality risk grade, using developmental and physical characteristics and degree of nourishment: the groups describe averagely developed and nourished neonates, those who were born with more or less overweight or weight deficit, as well as proportionally over- and underdeveloped newborns.

Having evaluated nearly 700,000 cases of Hungarian neonate data we have found that significant deviation from average physical development and nourishment - particularly undernourishment (disproportional retardation), extreme overnourishment and proportional retardation - is of great danger to both foetuses in utero and live-born neonates. This is valid for preterm and full-term foetuses, and for neonates as well.

As seen in Figure 2, undernourished (N = -3, -4, -5), or disproportionally-retarded, newborns can occur also above weight zone W2, above the 10th percentile. This is why the authors do not agree with the definition of retardation as those under the 10th percentile. Therefore, the authors offer a novel method to identify and differentiate proportionally retarded, disproportionally retarded and mixed type retarded newborns below the 10th weight percentile, as well as disproportionally retarded newborns over the 10th weight percentile. We should however mention that the MDN system is not suitable for determination of the genetically affected among the proportionally small newborns or for those who stayed proportionally small due to some pathological pregnancy reasons.

Our investigation found that if bodily development and nutrition significantly differ from the average, then the fetus has a significantly higher chance of intrauterine death, and this is also true for the newborn in the 1st-28th day of life. In this respect, the group of extremely disproportionally retarded is most at risk, followed by the extremely overnourished and the proportionally retarded, especially when extremely proportionally retarded. However, the proportionally overdeveloped fetuses and newborns are highly vulnerable as well.

In addition, the authors propose a definition expansion of the worldwide used concept of "perinatal mortality" concept. They further recommend the implementation of an "extended perinatal mortality" (EPM) definition along with obligatory differentiation of intrauterine mortality (IUM), and neonatal mortality of the live-born respectively (NM, 1st-28th day). This will allow weaknesses and strengths in prepartum, intrapartum and postpartum medical care to be identified.

The MDN system as a method can be applied in any country. Ideally, the development of neonates born in the studied country should be determined first according to country-specific (or preferably race-specific) weight and length percentile standards. Then, each neonate will be rated by and positioned in its nation-specific MDN matrix. The morbidity and mortality rates of different national neonate groups with equivalent positions in their national MDN matrices can be compared with this method. This also makes possible the comparison of neonatal morbidity and mortality data of countries, even if average birth weights are significantly different. The MDN system offers a tool to make more accurate and more reliable national and international comparative studies.

Such comparative studies have not really been realisable yet. So far, only the mortality of newborns with equal bodyweight has been compared, which makes little sense. Consider: is it possible to compare the chances of, say, a newborn in Papua New Guinea weighing 2, 400 grams with those of a newborn of 2,400 grams born in Norway? The body weight of 2,400 grams for a Papua New Guinea child corresponds to the national average birth standard, while its Norwegian counterpart corresponds to the weight of a premature infant, since in Norway the average full-term weight is 3,450 grams. A comparison like this obviously makes no sense. The implementation of the MDN system, however, solves this problem. If all countries would prepare national new-born weight and length standards, and each of the country's newborns would be placed in the locally relevant MDN matrix, national mortality and morbidity data of the same MDN population variations of newborns could be realistically compared. Such comparative studies would provide a more solid basis for scientific conclusions in comparison to those, made today based only on comparative weight tests. This is the supreme virtue of the MDN system, as this offers a tool to perform accurate national and international comparative studies.

The MDN system has another important area of application. It allows the prompt and accurate identification of those newborns for whom systematic follow-up measurements and growth hormone therapy treatment is likely to be necessary in the future. By positioning newborns in a corresponding area of the MDN matrix in the delivery room an immediate in situ distinction of proportional and mixed type retardation is possible. This is important because the mixed retarded group is the one with a later increased risk of certain diseases (hypertension, diabetes mellitus, etc). and therefore requires intensified observation. It is of great importance to register and follow up on the proportionally retarded and those with mixed retardation, for as a consequence they are most likely to lag behind the average growth rate in the future, and possibly require growth hormone treatment at the ages of 2-4.

In recent years enhanced interest in the MDN system gives us reason to hope that we have succeeded in enpowering the science and systematics of perinatology and pediatrics with a multifunctional, practical diagnostic tool.

6. References

Abernathy, JR., Greenberg BG., & Donelly JF. (1996). Birthweight, gestation and crownheel length, as response variable in multivariate analysis. *Am J Public Health,* 56, pp. 1281-1286.

Bakketeig, LS. (1998). Current growth standards, definitons, diagnosis and classification on fetal growth retardation. *Eur J Clin Nutr.* 52 (suppl 1), pp. 1-4.

Barker, DJP., Gluckman, PD., Goldfrey, KM., Harding, J., Owens, JA., & Robinson, JS. (1993). Fetal nutrition and adult disease. *Lancet,* 341, pp. 938-941.

Battaglia, FC., Lubchenco LO. (1967). A practical classification of newborn infants by weight and gestation age. *Pediatrics,* 71, pp. 159-170

Berkő, P. (1992). A study of the incidence, causes and consequences of retardation with the MDN system (*Thesis),* Miskolc

Berkő, P. (1996). The MDN system: A new concept and method for screening of IUGR (Abstract). *Prenat Neonat Med,* (suppl 1), pp. 331.

Berkő, P. (2006) A proposed new interpretation and revised definition of perinatal mortality. *Orv Hetil,* 147(6), pp. 269-274.

Berkő, P., Joubert, K. (2006). The effect of intrauterine development and nutritional status on intrauterine and neonatal mortality. *Orv.Hetil,* 147(29), pp. 1369-1375.

Berkő, P., Joubert K. (2009). The effect of intrauterine development and nutritional status on perinatal mortality. *J Matern Fetal Neonatal Med,* 22(7), pp. 552-559.

Deorari, AK., Aggarwal, R., & Paul, VK. (2001). Management of infants with intra-uterine growth restriction. *Indian J pediatr,* 68(12), pp.1155-1157.

Doszpod, J. (ed), (2000). *The intrauterine fetus,* Medicina, Budapest

Gyenis, Gy., Joubert, K., Klein, S., & Klein, B. (2004). Relationship among body height, socio-economic factors and mental abilities in Hungarian conscripts. *Anthrop Közl,* 45, pp. 165-172.

Gross, TL., Sokol, RJ. (eds.). (1989). *Intrauterine growth retardation.* Year Book Medical Publishers Inc, Chicago

Goldfrey, KM., Barker, DJP. (2000). Fetal nutrition and adult disease. *Am J. Clinical Nutrition,* 71, pp. 1344-1352.

Gruenwald, P. (1963). Chronic fetal distress and placental insufficiency. *Biol Neonate,* 5, pp. 215-221.

Gruenwald, P. (1966). Growth of the human fetus: I. Normal growth and its variations. *Am. J Obstet Gynec,* 94, pp. 1112-1121.

Henriksen, T. (1999). Foetal nutrition, foetal growth restriction and health later in life. *Acta Pediatr* (Suppl), 88(429), pp.4-8.

Joubert, K., Gyenis, Gy. (2003). Prenatal effects of intrauterine growth retardation on adult height of conscripts from Hungary. *HOMO Journal of Comparative Human Biology,* 54/2, pp. 104-112.

Joubert, K. (2000). Standards of birth weight and length based on liveborn data in Hungary, 1990-1996. *J Hungarian Gynecology,* 63, pp. 155-163.

Kady, MS., Gardosi, J. (2004). Prenatal mortality and fetal growth restriction. *Best Pract Res Clin Obstet Gynaecol,* 18 (3), pp. 397-410.

Kramer, MS., Olivier, M., McLean, FH., Dougherty, GE., Willis, DM., & Usher, RH. (1990). Determinants of Fetal Growth and Body Proportionality. *Pediatrics,* 86, pp. 18-26.

Kurjak, A., Latin,V., & Polak, J. (1978). Ultrasonic recognition of two types of growth retardation by measurment of four fetal dimensions. *J Perinat Med,* 6, pp. 102-108.

Lin, CC., Su, SJ. (1991). Comparison of associated high risk factors and perinatal outcome between symmetric and asymmetric fetal intrauterine growth retardation. *Am J Obstet Gynec,* 164, pp. 1535-1540.

Lin, CC. (1998). Current concepts of fetal growth restriction. *Obstet Gynec,* 92, pp. 1044-1049.

Lubchenco, LO., Hausmann, C., Dressler, M., & Boy, E. (1963). Intrauterine growth as estimated from liveborn birth weight data at 24-42 weeks of gestation. *Pediatrics,* 32, pp. 793-799.

Macfarlene, A., Chalmers, I., & Adelstein, AM. (1980). The role of standardization in the interpretation of perinatal mortality rates. *Health Trends,* 12, pp. 45-51.

Meredith, H. (1970). Body weight at birth of viable human infants: a worldwide comparative treatise. *Hum Biol,* 42, pp. 217-264.

Miller, HC., Hassanein, K. (1971). Diagnosis of impaired fetal growth in newborn infants. *Pediatrics,* 48, pp. 511-518.

Osmond, C., Barker, DJ. (2000). Fetal, infant, and childhood growth are predictors of coronary heart disaease, diabetes, and hypertension in adult men and women. *Environ Health Perspect,* 108 (suppl 3), pp. 545-553.

Rohrer, R. (1961). Der Index der Körperfülle als Mass des Ernährungszustandes. *Munch Med Wochensch,* 68, pp. 580-588.

Rosso, P., Winick, M. (1974). Intrauterine growth retardation. A new systematic approach based on the clinical and biochemical characteristics of this condition. *J Perinat Med,* 2, pp. 147-160.

Senterre, J. (1989). Inrauterine growth retardation. *Nestlé Nutrition Workshop Series,* Vol 18, Raven Press Ltd, New York

Shrimpton, R. (2003). Preventing low birthweight and reduction of child mortality. *Trans R Soc Trop Med Hyg,* 97(1), pp. 39-42.

Wollmann, HA. (1998). Intrauterine growth restriction: definition and etiology. *Horm Res,* 49 (suppl 2), pp. 1-6.

WHO. (1961). Public health aspects of low birth weight. *WHO Technical Report,* Series No. 217, Geneva

WHO. (1970). The prevention of perinatal mortality and morbidity. *WHO Technical Report* Series No. 457, Geneva

Wilcox, A., Russell, JT. (1983). Birthweight and perinatal mortality: II. On weight-specific mortality. *Intern J Epidem,* 12, pp. 319-326.

Wilcox, A., Russell, I. (1990). Why small black infants have a lower mortality rate than small white infants: The case for population-specific standards for birth weight. *J Pediatrics,* 116, pp. 7-16.

Zadik, Z., Dimant, O., Zung, A., & Reifen, R. (2003). Small for gestaional age: towards 2004. *J Endocrinol Invest,* 26(11), pp. 1143-1150.

3

Current Trends in Perinatal Mortality in Developing Countries: Nigeria as a Case Study

Uchenna Onwudiegwu and Ibraheem Awowole
Obafemi Awolowo University, Ile-Ife
Nigeria

1. Introduction

On November 20, 1989, the United Nations General Assembly adopted the Convention on the Rights of the Child after about a decade of deliberations between major stakeholders, including other United Nations agencies and Heads of Government of member states as well as Non-Governmental organisations (United Nations, 1989). In the World Summit for Children, which held a year later in 1990, world leaders further affirmed the need to promote earliest possible ratification and implementation of the Convention on the Rights of the Child, work for optimal growth and development in childhood, devise methods to eradicate hunger and globally attack poverty among other commitments, irrespective of race, age, colour, language, religion, socio-economic class or other considerations (United Nations, 1990).

A decade later, following further attempts by the United Nations to boost child survival and optimal development, the Millennium Development Goals (MDGs) were introduced with one of them, the MDG 4 specifically dedicated to children while the others directly or indirectly promote it.

Perinatal mortality is simply one of the earliest indicators reflecting each countries effort at ensuring that these goals are actualised and that children are not only protected, but develop to their maximal potentials.

1.1 Definitions

Perinatal mortality is defined by the World Health Organization as the demise of a fetus in utero after the age of viability, during labour or within the first 7 days of extra-uterine life. Technically, this may be represented as Stillbirths + Early Neonatal deaths (WHO).

This definition allowed each country to supply its own data based on the nationally accepted age of viability in that country. This may result in loss of uniformity, thereby reducing the validity of international comparisons. While the World Health Organization, the International Stillbirth Alliance and some developed countries utilise 22 weeks as their age of viability (WHO, 2006). and may therefore report a loss at that gestational age as perinatal mortality, a country like Nigeria, with its age of viability as 28 weeks will simply report it as an abortion. For the purpose of eliminating ambiguity and ensuring uniformity, the World Health Organisation had gone ahead to define live birth and stillbirth clearly as follows (WHO, 2004);

"Live birth is the complete expulsion or extraction from its mother of a product of conception, irrespective of the duration of the pregnancy, which, after such separation, breathes or shows any other evidence of life, such as beating of the heart, pulsation of the umbilical cord, or definite movement of voluntary muscles, whether or not the umbilical cord has been cut or the placenta is attached" while a stillbirth on the other hand is defined as "death prior to the complete expulsion or extraction from its mother of a product of conception, irrespective of the duration of pregnancy; the death is indicated by the fact that after such separation the fetus does not breathe or show any other evidence of life, such as beating of the heart, pulsation of the umbilical cord or definite movement of voluntary muscles".

These definitions are therefore irrespective of gestational age. Despite this however, many countries continue to report perinatal mortality relative to gestational age.

Perinatal mortality rate moves a step further to evaluate the absolute number of perinatal deaths relative to the total number of births. It is usually expressed as an annual figure and it is calculated as (WHO, 2006);

$$\frac{\text{Stillbirths + Early Neonatal deaths}}{\text{Total births}} \text{ X } 1000$$

The use of Perinatal mortality rate had however been criticised because many countries still report it based on their age of viability as stated earlier. Another criticism against it is that many developing countries either have incomplete or completely lack information on useful parameters such as stillbirth rates, necessitating estimation and extrapolation of National figures from surveys. This may make it grossly under-reported and inaccurate. It is however saddening that despite these disparities; developing countries still have perinatal mortality rates that are many folds of that reported by the developed countries.

Another challenge in the utilisation of perinatal mortality as an index of assessing health care status is that it completely ignores the birth weight of the newborn. It is also completely silent on the causes of death and therefore cannot be used solely on its own merit as a tool based on which specific measures will be planned. Despite these criticisms however, perinatal mortality rates still have the peculiar advantage of taking into consideration stillbirth rates, a very important index in maternal and newborn health care that even the Millennium Development Goals targets and indicators ignored. Specifically, it is an important indicator of the quality of obstetric and paediatric care available in any setting.

In an attempt to complement the utilisation of perinatal mortality rate, many classification systems had been put forward, such that each country can then review the causes of death in the perinatal period and institute local measures to tackle it appropriately. Some of these classification systems include; the Wigglesworth classification, Tulip classification, Whitfield classification, ReCoDe, CoDaC and the modified Whitfield classification systems (Froen et al, 2009; Gardosi et al, 2005; Korteweg et al, 2006; Chan et al, 2006; Whitfield et al, 1986; Wigglesworth et al, 1980).

The magnitude of innocent lives lost in the transition and early adaptation period to life is colossal. About 133 million babies are born alive each year with over 6.3 million perinatal deaths occurring worldwide. Of these perinatal deaths, 3.3 million are stillbirths while 3 million deaths occur in the first week of life (WHO, 2006). A total of 3.7 million deaths, accounting for almost 40% of under-five deaths occur in the neonatal period. This simply means that as much as 75% of neonatal deaths occur in the first week of life (early neonatal period)(WHO, 2004), an additional signal to the strength in perinatal mortality as an index for monitoring health care status. With 98% of these deaths occurring in developing countries and 27% in the least developed countries (Stanton et al, 2006), perinatal mortality in developing countries is obviously receiving far too little attention. Worse still, for every newborn baby that dies, at least another twenty newborns suffer birth injuries, complications arising from preterm birth or other neonatal conditions (Unicef, 2009).

2. Nigeria as a case study

Nigeria was chosen for this review because it is simply Africa's most populous country with about 150 million citizens. The country with a total fertility rate of 5.2 readily records over 6 million births annually (Unicef, 2009) and despite being just about 2% of the global population, contributes significantly to the perinatal, neonatal and under five mortality in the world. It is not surprising that Nigeria, with its buoyant population and high mortality rates single-handedly contributes about 8% of the world's annual mortality in neonates with an annual figure of 242,000 neonates' death (WHO, 2006; Federal Ministry of Health, Nigeria, 2011), a feat for which the country comfortably leads the neonatal mortality chart in Africa (Lawn at al, 2010). The country, despite a per capital income of 1140 dollars and an annual growth rate of 1.7% in the last 20 years (Unicef, 2009) had an under-five mortality rate of 230 per 1,000 live births in 1990, 207 per 1,000 live births in 2000 and 186 per 1,000 live births in 2009 (WHO, 2010) and is currently ranked 18th on the under-5 mortality list (Unicef, 2009). With this scenario, Nigeria amazingly records a total under-five death of almost a million annually (Cousens et al, 2010).

The World Health Organization estimated perinatal deaths in Nigeria to be about 30 per 1000 live births in 1990, only for this figure to increase almost three-folds ten years later. This can be attributed to the short and long term consequences of the depressed economy of the country within this period, which became marked from about five years earlier - 1985. This led to the introduction of an economic revival programme under the acronym 'Structural Adjustment Programme' (SAP) by the Federal Government; a programme that led to partial and in some situations to the outright withdrawal of health subsidies in the country, leading to a rapid decline in the utilisation of maternal health services (Onwudiegwu, 1993, 1997). This high level of perinatal mortality in Nigeria means that the country's dream of achieving MDG-4 by the year 2015 may after all be a mirage unless decisive steps are taken.

At a national level, countries like Finland recorded the lowest stillbirth rate of 2.0 per 1000 births while Nigeria ranked second only behind Pakistan with a national stillbirth rate of 42 per 1000 deliveries. Nigeria is also among the top ten countries which together contribute 54% of total world births and unfortunately also account for 67% of all stillbirths (WHO, 2010).

Indigenous hospital-based reviews from the Northern part of Nigeria in 1993 reported a perinatal mortality rate of 58.6 per 1000 deliveries. The same study however reported an age-specific perinatal mortality rate of 375 per 1000 births among teenage mothers with birth trauma being the leading cause of perinatal death (Akpala, 1993). This study not only revealed the high perinatal mortality rate but also confirmed the significant contribution of teenage pregnancy to perinatal mortality. Nigeria's perinatal mortality rate may perhaps not be so surprising, considering the fact that the country has an adolescent fertility rate of 126 per 1,000 girls aged 15-19 years (WHO, 2010).

A five year retrospective study at the University of Nigeria Teaching Hospital, Enugu, south eastern Nigeria, between the periods of 1995 and the year 2000 (Adimora and Odetunde, 2007) revealed a perinatal mortality rate of 133.94 per 1,000 births, an unacceptably high rate while another study by Kuti et al (2003) at Obafemi Awolowo University Teaching Hospital, Ile-Ife, South-Western Nigeria, in the succeeding 5 year period between 1996 to 2000 reported a perinatal mortality rate of 77.03 per 1000 total births. This study also went on to report the causes of these deaths with asphyxia, accounting for 58% being the commonest cause. Other significant causes include prematurity and early neonatal infections. The high incidence of unbooked patients, multiple pregnancies and low birth weight babies were cited as major contributors to the high perinatal mortality rates in our environment.

Onwudiegwu (1994) on the other hand took a community-based approach to the challenges of perinatal mortality, and factors such as formal educational status of women, rural/urban dwelling, birth interval and birth order were the significant contributors identified in South-Western part of the country. Contrary to the academic causes of these deaths however, a critical evaluation revealed that the problems that contribute to perinatal mortality in Nigeria as well as other developing countries go way beyond the identified medical causes.

Some of these causes are peculiar to the policies in the country while others simply relate to the health of the mothers and their attitudes. In a country where 58% of pregnant women had only one antenatal clinic attendance and even fewer women (45%) had at least four clinic visits (Unicef , 2009; WHO, 2010), the effect is of course poor maternal and perinatal outcome. Even more worrisome as expressed by Onwudiegwu (1994) is the fact that a proportion of women who despite having received antenatal care in the hospital resorted to delivery in the traditional settings or spiritual homes because of economic or spiritual reasons, while some simply stated disapproval by their husbands as their excuse.

The contraceptive prevalence in the country is also at an unbelievably low level of 15% in 2009, about 50% less than the contraceptive utilisation prevalence in the neighbouring country Cameroun (WHO, 2010; National population commission 2008). This ultimately results in high fertility rates and reduction in birth interval with the overall effect manifesting as high fetal wastages.

2.1 What about the mothers?

It is very difficult and extremely negligent to consider perinatal health without relating it to the state of health of mothers. This is another benefit that the use of perinatal mortality confers as it not only considers the babies but also reflects the state of health of the mothers delivering them as well. Women in developing countries generally tend to have many pregnancies. Their lifetime risk of dying in pregnancy therefore reflects the overall burden on these women. Nigeria, with a maternal mortality ratio (WHO, 2010) of 1,100 per 100,000 is one of the fourteen countries worldwide with a maternal mortality ratio of at least 1000 per 100,000 deliveries. A woman's lifetime risk of dying in pregnancy in developing countries is many folds that of the developed countries but the difference is more marked when countries like Nigeria with a 1 in 18 maternal risk of dying is compared with 1 in 48,000 for Ireland! (WHO, 2007). With Nigeria recording a staggering 33,000 maternal deaths each year and with about 4 stillborns and seven newborns dying for each maternal death, the perinatal mortality rate in the country is not so surprising after all (Federal Ministry of Health, 2011, WHO, UNFPA, 2010).

The health status of the mother and that of the newborn are very intimately related: death of the mother automatically spells doom for those newborns that are fortunate enough to survive the condition that caused the demise of the mother. With so many women dying in pregnancy in Nigeria, the resulting colossal effect on perinatal mortality cannot be overemphasized. Complications during birth, such as obstructed and prolonged labour are established risks for perinatal mortality, yet they are common sights in our everyday practice. Current obstetric practices such as the use of partographs in monitoring labour had proven so effective in preventing these conditions (Orji et al, 2007; Fatusi et al, 2008), yet, this simple and inexpensive practice eludes many Nigerian parturients.

Lack of maternal health care is causing a large proportion of perinatal deaths by two unique mechanisms other than the commonly listed medical causes of perinatal mortality. These include the deaths resulting as a complication of the condition that killed the mother and the second one is lack of maternal care for the newborn post partum owing to the death of the mother.

Intrapartum death rate is a very important indicator enabling health personnel to take the most appropriate measures to prevent such deaths. An estimated 24- 37% of babies born as stillbirths in developing countries actually die intrapartum. In Nigeria, intrapartum fetal death is estimated to be about 25% (FMOH, 2011). The main factors responsible for these intrapartum deaths are simply poor maternal health, suboptimal care during pregnancy and medical conditions which had not been diagnosed or was inappropriately treated before or during pregnancy, coupled with the peculiarity of the travails of a pregnant woman labouring in Nigeria where only 39% of them benefit from skilled attendance at delivery and 35% actually had institutionalised deliveries (Unicef, 2009; National Population Commission, 2008). In women who receive good care during childbirth, intrapartum deaths are due to unexpected severe obstetric complications and it accounts for less than 10% of stillbirths (WHO, 2003).

The intrapartum deaths are directly related to the place of delivery, which is at home in about 62% of cases in Nigeria and this also reflects why many of these cases may not be reported, while delivery in health facilities were reported in only 35% of cases (FMOH, 2011; NPC, 2008). Even some of workers in these health facilities lack appropriate knowledge in the use of partograph for monitoring the progress of labour (Orji et al, 2007; Fatusi et al, 2008).

The "three delays" model (Thaddeus and Maine, 1994) can also be adapted to explain the high proportion of intrapartum deaths, either singly or in combination. Onwudiegwu et al

(1999) identified type 3 delay as an important contributor to perinatal and maternal mortality and went on to report a mean decision-caesarean delivery interval of four hours in women with indications for emergency caesarean section as a cause of some of the perinatal deaths. Another report (Omo-Aghoja et al, 2010) from Benin, South-South Nigeria also identified associated type three delay in 61.9% of the maternal deaths. Type three delay could not be better exemplified!

The major contributors to maternal mortality in Nigeria include haemorrhage (23%), infection (17%), unsafe abortion (11%), obstructed labour (11%), eclampsia/hypertensive disorders of pregnancy (11%), malaria (11%) and anaemia (11%) (FMOH, 2007). All these are causes that could readily be taken care of by a well co-ordinated Emergency Obstetric Care (EmOC), a collection of services with the aim of reducing maternal mortality by improving the availability, accessibility, quality and use of services for the treatment of complications that arise during pregnancy and childbirth. The recommendation of this programme is to ensure at least five EmOC facilities, including at least one comprehensive facility per 500 000 population. Seven services are expected to be rendered by the Basic EmOC facilities while the Comprehensive centres will render additional two services to make a total of nine (WHO, UNICEF et al, 2009). The unfortunate challenge in many countries however is that many of these facilities, albeit established, were not functioning. In Nigeria, a random survey of 12 out of the 36 states in the country revealed that only 4.2% of the available public facilities in those states met the criteria for EmOC! (Fatusi and Ijadunola, 2003).

Nigeria's health status definitely appears deplorable from all the aforementioned but things would have been worse than they are if the Government, Non Governmental organisations and individual stakeholders in the country had not been taking active and drastic measures to combat the trend. These are the reasons why the under- five mortality rate declined by 22% between the five year period of 2003 and 2008 (NPC , 2008).

The urban-rural dissociation in health care is perhaps best demonstrated in no other country than Nigeria. Factors such as teenage pregnancies, lack of health care facilities and human resources are extremely common in these rural areas where as stated earlier, at least 51% of Nigerians reside (Unicef, 2009). Presently, despite the associated adverse outcome, 29% of teenage girls aged 15-19years are married and at least 28% of them reported giving birth to their first child before the age of 18 years, most of these in rural areas (Unicef, 2009; NPC, 2008).

The Society of Obstetrics and Gynaecology of Nigeria further supported this by reporting an all time high maternal mortality ratio of 7, 523 per 100,000 deliveries in Kano, a rural state in Northern Nigeria (Society of Gynaecology and Obstetrics of Nigeria, 2004).

In an attempt to promote improvement in equity and access to care, the Nigerian Midwives Service Scheme (MSS) was introduced. Women who deliver in rural areas have been documented to have an increased risk of perinatal mortality and other adverse outcome in pregnancy compared with their counterparts in urban areas, yet 51% of Nigeria's population live in the rural communities. In order to bridge the gap of human resources and improve the health status of rural community dwellers, the Federal Government initiated this programme which involves deploying newly qualified, unemployed and retired midwives to rural areas to render their services after they had been trained to proficiency in basic obstetrics life saving skills and integrated management of childhood illnesses. The programme is currently recording great success in the country (FMOH, 2011).

Contraceptive usage, though universally agreed to be at a lower prevalence rate in Nigeria than the regional average has also definitely impacted some benefits and that probably account for the progressive fall in total fertility rate in Nigeria from 6.6, where it had remained stagnant for the 20 year period preceding 1990 to the present figure of 5.7 (FMOH, 2011; NPC, 2008).. It is expected that with progressive fall in the number of children a woman delivers, the total burden of morbidity and the cumulative risk of dying from the reproductive process also reduces.

At the local level, people are also making efforts to ensure a safe transition from in utero to life for these newborn by intensifying efforts at reducing the burden of intrapartum deaths from obstructed and prolonged labour by educating health workers on the partographic monitoring of labour. The benefit from this was clearly demonstrated in South west Nigeria where training programmes conducted on the use of partographs in labour resulted in a significant reduction in perinatal mortality (Orji et al, 2007; Fatusi et al, 2008).

Poverty was identified as the main barrier to accessing health services in about 56% of Nigerian women in 2008 (NPC, Nigeria, 2008). Poverty alone could not have been responsible for the ordeals in Nigeria as other countries in Sub-Saharan Africa who are not as wealthy as Nigeria, including Botswana, Eritrea and Malawi are already adjudged to be on track to achieving MDG 4. Nigeria on the other hand had recorded an average annual reduction rate of 1.2% and presently needs a miraculous 10% annual reduction if it is to meet the two-third reduction in under-five mortality by the year 2015 (FMOH, 2011)

The country is wealthier on the average than these other countries in Africa with better indices, some of whom are even adjudged to be on track to achieving the health related MDGs. The country is just yet to commit and co-ordinate its human and material resources in adequate proportions to this course. In 2001, the country pledged to progressively increase budgetary allocations to health. This increment in budgetary allocation has improved minimally from less than 5% to its present rate of 6.5%,[16] which is not sufficient to achieve its goals. In a bid to sustain this however, the country further affirm its commitment at the last United Nations Summit held in New York in September 2010, pledging to increase its budgetary allocation to health to as much as 15% by 2015 (United Nations, 2010). This is a most welcome development.

The Birth, Death compulsory registration decree was established in 1992 in order to establish a child's legal status and enhance the appropriate planning and provision for such children by producing a formidable data base. Presently however, only about 30% of live births in Nigeria are registered, with deliveries in urban areas being twice as likely to be registered compared with rural settings (Unicef, 2009; FMOH, 2011; NPC, 2008). Stillbirths, majority of which occur at home are even less likely to be reported. This ultimately deprives the country of appropriate and accurate data for planning. It is advised that the Government and citizens of the country make extra effort to report these vital statistics.

A woman's educational status goes a long way in influencing her health seeking behaviour and this reflects most in no other place than perinatal, neonatal and maternal mortality. These indices decline by about 50% or more as the woman's educational status increases.

This has been explained by the fact that she is likely to delay her marriage, use contraception and health services appropriately as well as utilise her knowledge to establish the best rational decisions for herself and her family members. Nigeria, with a net female primary and secondary school enrolment ratio (Unicef, 2009) of 58% and 33% respectively definitely has a long way to go if the country hopes to adopt female education as one of its strategies to reduce perinatal mortality. Promoting education of the girl child to at least secondary school level is therefore recommended for the countries administrators.

Lastly, HIV/AIDS has been a most unfair burden on the country. 1.8 percent of the population of Nigeria was infected with HIV in 1991. Subsequent reports revealed HIV prevalence rates of 3.8% in 1993, 4.5% in 1998 and presently 3.6% of the Nigerian population have the disease (Unicef, 2009; UNGASS, 2010). This prevalence may appear low compared to what obtains in other African countries but considering the large population of Nigeria, the absolute number of people affected is actually enormous, translating to 3.3 million individuals. Out of this figure, 1.7 million are women and as much as 360,000 children are aged 0-4 years. Currently, the World Health organization reported that 6.2% of maternal deaths are directly attributable to HIV/AIDS in Africa (Khan, 2006). Various efforts by the Nigerian Government in response to this challenge include the formation of The President's Committee on AIDS (PCA) in 1999 and the National Action Committee on AIDS (NACA) in the year 2000. Further efforts include the establishment of a three-year HIV/AIDS Emergency Action Plan (HEAP). Presently, a National strategic framework that will span a period of 5 years (2010-2015) is being executed as one of the activities of NACA (National Agency for Control of AIDS, 2009). Nigeria currently also benefits from partnering with other donor agencies such as the President's Emergency Plan for AIDS Relief (PEPFAR), Global Funds and the World Bank.

3. Conclusion

Finally, it is essential to state that there is no short-cut to the desired improvement in perinatal mortality rates for Nigeria and other developing countries. Nigeria has been used as a case study in this article, but the situation is not so different in many developing countries. The identified medical and socio-economic causes of perinatal mortality are closely linked to the causes of maternal mortality. Developing countries are therefore encouraged to desist from merely being attendees at International Summits and signatories to all United Nations declarations to actually executing the recommendations at their homestead. The recent introduction of the Integrated Maternal, Newborn and Child Health (IMNCH) strategy, an accelerated plan of action which aims to provide a continuum of care for mothers, newborns and children in a single package while ensuring universal coverage of these interventions by the Federal Ministry of Health of Nigeria is a welcome idea in this direction (FMOH, 2007). The Millennium Development Goals are feasible, but only with adequate mobilization, sustained dedication and commitments of material and human resources to the cause of our women and newborns. The Millennium Development Goals are not invincible!

4. References

Akpala CO. Perinatal mortality in northern Nigeria rural community. J Roy Soc Prom Health. 1993;113(3):124-127.

Chan A, King JF, Flenady V, Haslam RH, Tudehope DI. Classification of perinatal deaths: development of the Australian and New Zealand classifications. J Paediatr Child Health. 2004;40(7):340-347.

Cousens S, Blencowe H, Stanton S, Chou D, Ahmed S, Steinhardt L, et al. National, regional, and worldwide estimates of stillbirth rates in 2009 with trends since 1995: a systematic analysis. Lancet. 2011;377.

Fatusi AO, Ijadunola KT. National Study on Essential Obstetric Care Facilities in Nigeria. Abuja, Federal Ministry of Health & United Nations Population Fund (UNFPA); 2003.

Fatusi AO, Makinde ON, Adeyemi AB, Orji EO, Onwudiegwu U. Evaluation of health workers' training in use of the partogram. Int Journal Gynecol Obstet. 2008;100:41-44.

Federal Ministry of Health. Integrated Maternal, Newborn and Child Health Strategy. Abuja; 2007.

Federal Ministry of Health. Saving newborn lives in Nigeria: Newborn health in the context of the Integrated Maternal, Newborn and Child Health Strategy. 2nd ed. Abuja. : Federal Ministry of Health, Save the Children, Jhpiego; 2011.

Frøen JF, Pinar H, Flenady V, Bahrin S, Charles A, Chauke L, et al. Causes of death and associated conditions (Codac) - a utilitarian approach to the classification of perinatal deaths. BMC Pregnancy and Childbirth. 2009;9:22.

Gardosi J, Kady SM, McGeown P, Francis A, Tonks A. Classification of stillbirth by relevant condition at death (ReCoDe): population based cohort study. BMJ. 2005;331:1113.

GN Adimora, IO Odetunde. Perinatal mortality in University of Nigeria Teaching Hospitan (UNTH) Enugu at the end of the last millenium. Nig J Clin Pract. 2007;10(1):19-23.

Korteweg FJ, Gordijn SJ, Timmer A, Erwich JJ, Bergman KA, Bouman K, et al. The Tulip classification of perinatal mortality: introduction and multidisciplinary inter-rater agreement. BJOG. 2006;113(4):393-401.

Kuti O, Orji EO, Ogunlola IO. Analysis of perinatal mortality in a Nigerian teaching hospital. J Obstet Gynaecol. 2003;23(5):512-514.

Khan KS. WHO analysis of causes of maternal death: a systematic review. Lancet. 2006;367:1066-1074.

Lawn JE, Kerber K, Enweronu-Laryea C, Cousens S. 3.6 million neonatal deaths: what is progressing, what is not. Sem Perinatol 2010;1053:1-23.

Maternal mortality in 2005: estimates developed by WHO, UNICEF, UNFPA and the World Bank. Geneva WHO, 2007,.

National Population Commission. Nigeria Demographic and Health Survey 2008. Abuja: National Population Commission, Federal Republic of Nigeria, 2009

National Agency for the Control of AIDS (NACA). 'National HIV/AIDS strategic framework (NSF) 2010-15'. 2009.

Onwudiegwu U. The effect of a depressed economy on the utilisation of maternal health services: The Nigerian experience. J Obstet Gynaecol. 1993;13:311-314.

Onwudiegwu U. A Community Survey of Perinatal Mortality in South-Western Nigeria.: Takemi Programme in International Health,Harvard School of Public Health; 1994.

Onwudiegwu U. The effect of a depressed economy on the utilisation of maternal health services: The Nigerian experience II. J Obstet Gynaecol. 1997;17(2):143-148.

Onwudiegwu U, Makinde ON, Ezechi OC, Adeyemi AB. Decision-caesarean delivery interval in a Nigerian university hospital: implications for maternal morbidity and mortality. J Obstet Gynaecol. 1999;19(1):30-33.

Orji EO, Fatusi AA, Makinde ON, Adeyemi AB, Onwudiegwu U. Impact of Training on the Use of Partograph on Maternal and Perinatal Outcome in Peripheral Health Centers. J Turkish-German Gynecol Assoc. 2007;8(2):148-152.

Omo-Aghoja LO, Aisien OA, Akuse JT, Okonofua FE. Maternal mortality and emergency obstetric care in Benin City, South-south Nigeria. J Chin Clin Med. 2010;3(5):3.

Stanton C, Lawn JE, Rahman H, Wilczynska-Ketende K, Hill K. Stillbirth rates: delivering estimates in 190 countries. Lancet. 2006;367:1487-1494.

Society o f Gynecology and Obstetrics of Nigeria. Status of emergency obstetrics services for safe motherhood in six states of Nigeria: A project report submitted to the Macarthur Foundation, USA. 2004.

United Nations. Global strategy for women's and children's health: commitments summary. New York: United Nations 2010.

Thaddeus S, Maine D. Too far to walk: maternal mortality in context. Soc sci med. 1994;38:091-110.

United Nations. U.N. Convention on the Rights of the Child1989.

United Nations. World Declaration on the Survival, Protection and Development of Children and a Plan of Action1990.

Unicef. State of the World's Children 2009: Maternal and Newborn Health. Unicef 2009.

Unicef. At a glance: Nigeria: Unicef 2009.

World Health Organization. International statistical classification of diseases and related health problems. Geneva: World Health Organization, 2004.

WHO. Neonatal and perinatal mortality. country, regional and global estimates. Geneva: World Health Organization 2006.

Whitfield CR, Smith NC, Cockburn F, Gibson AA. Perinatally related wastage--a proposed classification of primary obstetric factors. Br J Obstet Gynaecol. 1986;93(7):694-703.

Wigglesworth JS. Monitoring perinatal mortality. A pathophysiological approach. Lancet. 1980;2(8196):684-686.

World Health Organization. Neonatal and Perinatal Mortality: Country, regional and global estimates. Geneva: WHO.2004.

WHO. World Health Statistics 2010. Geneva: WHO 2010.

WHO, UNFPA, The World Bank. Trends in maternal mortality: 1990-2008: World Health Organization. Geneva 2010.

WHO, Unicef, AMDD, UNFPA. Monitoring Emergency Obstetric Care; A Handbook: World Health Organization 2009.

UNGASS (2010). 'UNGASS Country Progress Report: Nigeria'.

4

Neonatal Mortality: Incidence, Correlates and Improvement Strategies

Sajjad ur Rahman[1,3] and Walid El Ansari[2,3]
[1]*Weill Cornell Medical College, Doha*
[2]*Faculty of Applied Sciences,*
University of Gloucestershire, Gloucester
[3]*Lead Principal Investigator PEARL Study**
[1]*State of Qatar*
[2]*United Kingdom*

1. Introduction

1.1 Aim

The current chapter provides a review of definitions, incidence, correlates and global magnitude of neonatal mortality. The chapter also presents evidence based strategies to improve neonatal survival particularly in resource constrained developing countries.

The neonatal period (birth to 28th day of life) is the most vulnerable and high-risk time in lifebecause of the highest mortality and morbidity incidence in human life during this period. An estimated 40percent of deaths in children less than five years of age occur during the first 28 days of life (WHO, 2011a). The remaining 60 percent of deaths occur during the subsequent 1800 days of the first five years of life. The average daily mortality rate during the neonatal period is close to 30 fold higher than during the postnatal period (one month to one year of age). During 2010, an estimated 7.7 million children under five years of age died worldwide (Rajaratnam et al., 2010). This included 3.1 million neonatal deaths, 2.3 million post neonatal deaths (age one month to one year) and 2.3 million childhood deaths (age 1-4 years).

The neonatal period is the extra uterine continuum of intrauterine foetal life separated by birth, which is the time when umbilical cord is severed. During the intrauterine period, foetal life is dependent on its connection with the uterus through the placenta and umbilical cord. The neonatal period is the beginning of an independent extra uterine life. The transition from foetal to neonatal life is usually very smooth in a full term newborn baby (37-41 weeks gestation), born through a normal uncomplicated vaginal delivery, which is the case in the vast majority of births. However, the process can be complicated either because of problems in the mother, foetus, placenta, environment, the procedures of birth, or any combination of these factors leading to neonatal mortality and / or morbidity. The neonatal mortality is not only a strong indicator of neonatal, perinatal and maternal health

---

*Perinatal Neonatal Outcomes Research Study in the Arabian Gulf (PEARL Study)

in any given country, region or population; it is also a very big challenge for the health strategists and perinatal health care planners.

2. Definitions

2.1 Neonatal, post neonatal and Infant mortality

In infants (age 0-364 days), the first 28 days of life (day 0 to day 27) after birth are known as neonatal period (WHO, 2011a), and day 28 to day 364 as post neonatal period (Rowley, 1994). The neonatal mortality rate (NMR) is defined as the number of neonatal deaths (during the first 28 completed days of life) per one thousand live births in a given year or other period (WHO, 2011b). The Post Neonatal Mortality Rate (PNMR) is defined as the number of post neonatal deaths (from day 28 of life till the first birth day) per one thousand live births per year or other given period (WHO, 2011b). The Neonatal and Post neonatal mortality together constitutes the Infant Mortality which is defined as the number of infant deaths from birth to one year of age per 1000 live births during the same period. Infant Mortality Rate (IMR) is a very strong indicator of child health in a country, region or population and is used as a yard stick of progress in health care improvement.

2.2 Early and late neonatal mortality

The neonatal period is further sub-divided into early and late neonatal periods (WHO, 2011b). Early neonatal period corresponds to the first seven completed days of life (day 0 to 6) while the late neonatal period lasts from day 7 to day 27. The majority of problems during the early neonatal period are causally related with the foetal life or the birth process; while most problems during late neonatal life are acquired. Early Neonatal Mortality Rate (ENMR) is defined as the number of neonatal deaths during the first seven days of life per 1000 live births in a given year or any other period. Late Neonatal Mortality Rate (LNMR) is defined as the number of neonatal deaths between day seven and day 27 of life per 1000 live births in a given year or any other period. Most neonatal deaths occur during early neonatal period. Globally some three quarters of neonatal deaths happen in the first week after birth (Zupan & Aahman, 2005). In Europe the early neonatal deaths range from 58 percent (Czech Republic) to 89 percent (Northern Ireland) (Euro-Peristat, 2008). The ENMR in Europe is 1.5 to 3.8 and the LNMR is 0.3 to 1.9 per one thousand live births (Fig. 1).

Within the Early neonatal period, mortality is highest (25-45 percent) on day one of life (Lawn et al., 2005) and decreases as the age advances in number of days (Fig. 2). The Euro-Peristat project (2008) reported a trend of shifting mortality from early to late neonatal period among European countries. This is probably because of better and improved perinatal care for very sick babies at the time of birth and immediate postnatal period.

2.3 Perinatal mortality

The intrauterine foetal period, in combination with early neonatal period is called Perinatal period. Therefore, combined foetal and early neonatal deaths constitute Perinatal Mortality. Foetal death before or during birth (antepartum or intra partum respectively) is also designated as still birth. Foetal deaths in the second trimester (< 28 weeks gestation) are designated as early foetal deaths while foetal deaths in third trimester (≥ 28 weeks gestation) are designated as late foetal deaths (Fig 3). Perinatal Mortality Rate (PMR) is defined as a sum of still births (foetal deaths) and early neonatal deaths in a given period of time per 1000 total live plus still births during the same period in the same population. Since the definition of foetal period varies in individual countries, ranging from 16 to 28 weeks of gestation, the definition of Perinatal Period also varies from country to country (Euro-Peristat Project, 2008).

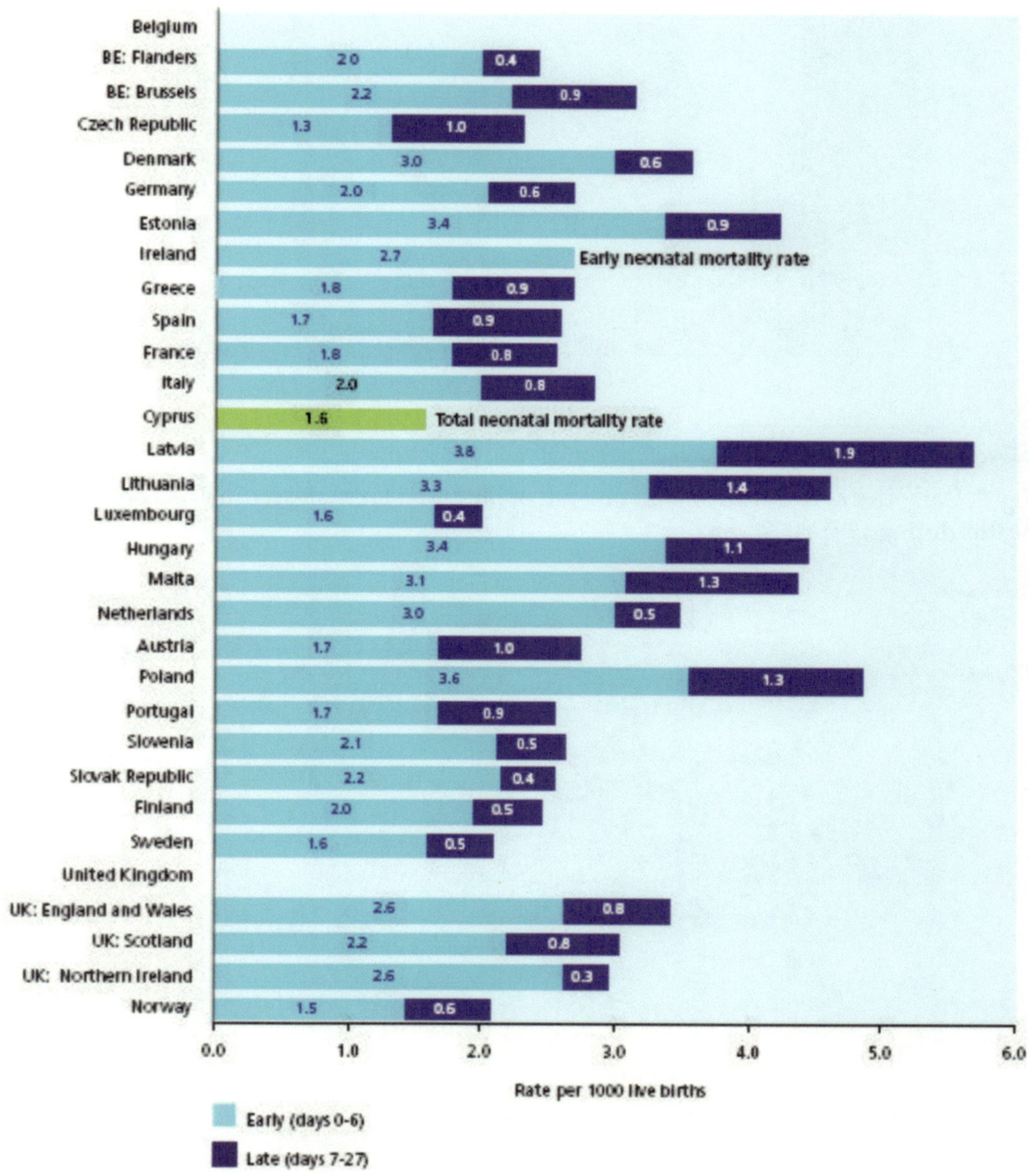

Source: Euro-Peristat 2008, with permission of the Europeristat Project Team

Fig. 1. Early and Late Neonatal Mortality Rates among European countries.

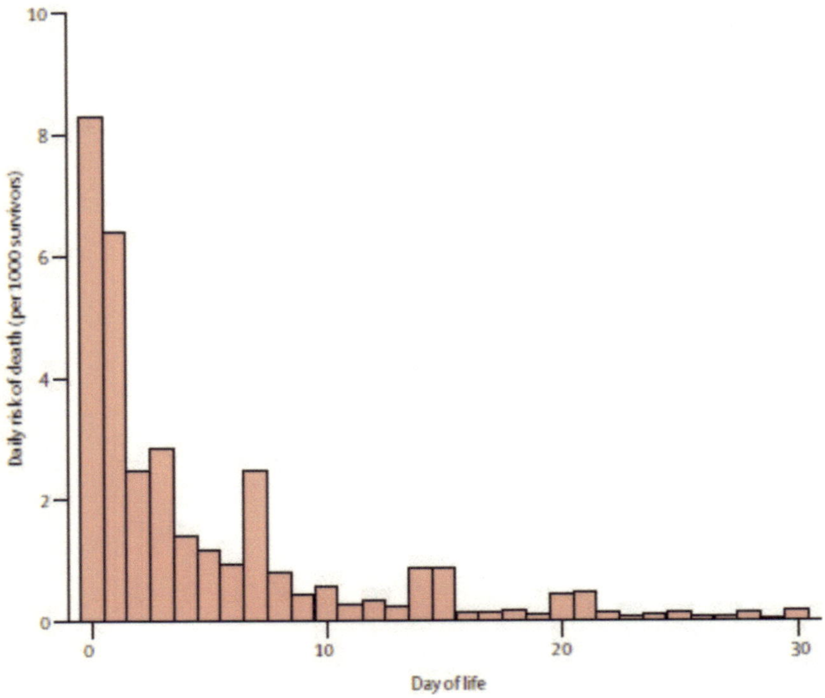

Source: Lawn, 2005 with permission of the authors and publishers

Fig. 2. Daily risk of death during first month of life based on analysis of 10048 neonatal deaths during 1995-2003.

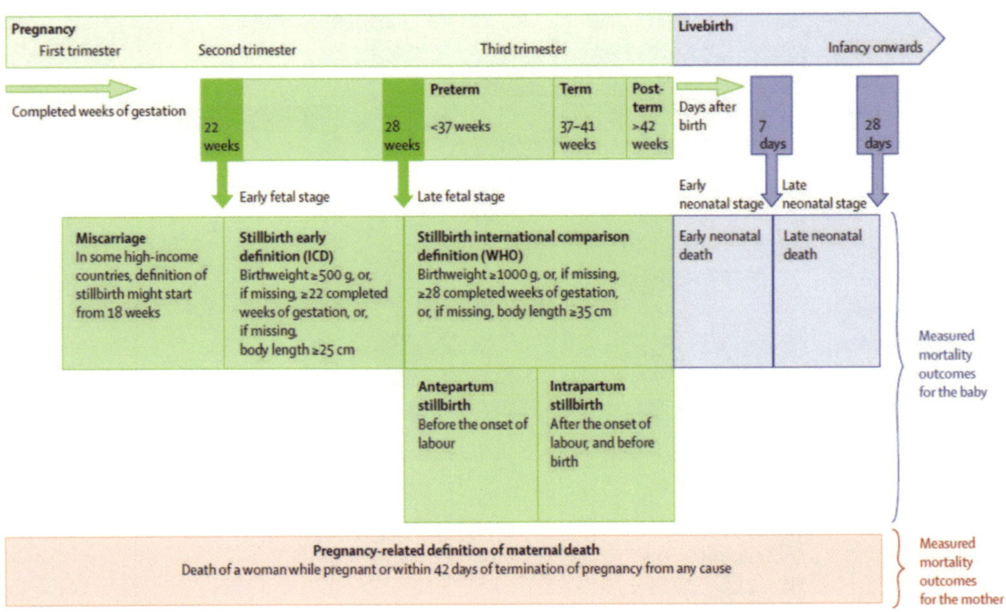

Source: Lawn, J E. (2011)

Fig. 3. Maternal, Fetal, Neonatal and Perinatal Mortality during and after Pregnancy.

The International Classification of Diseases 10th revision (ICD-10), by WHO, defines foetal deaths using one of the three criteria in the following order; a birth weight of 500 grams or more; if birth weight is unknown, a gestational age of 22 weeks or more; and if both these criteria are unknown, a crown heel length of 25 cm or more. In some countries e.g. Australia, not only the foetal period is extended down to 20 weeks gestation and 400 grams birth weight; the perinatal period is also extended by including the whole neonatal period (day 0-27) instead of early neonatal period (Australian Bureau of Statistics 2009). These variations make inter country and regional comparisons of still birth rate and perinatal mortality rates very difficult. Therefore, for international comparisons, WHO recommends reporting of late foetal deaths (third trimester stillbirths at ≥ 1000 grams birth weight, ≥ 28 weeks gestation, ≥ 35 cm body length). PMR, in association with Maternal, Foetal and Neonatal Mortality Rates, is a very strong indicator of Maternal and Newborn care in any country /population (Fig 3).

3. Neonatal mortality: The global magnitude of the problem in 2011

The 2010 toll of global neonatal deaths ranges from 3.1 million per year (Rajaratnam, 2010) to 3.4 million per year (Population Reference Bureau, 2010). These estimates are based on varying data collection tools and statistical methods. Table1 shows that, of the 140 million babies born worldwide, 90percent were born in low-income countries and 10% in high-income countries while approximately 99percent of neonatal deaths occur in low income countries and 1percent in high income countries. Every minute seven newborn babies die worldwide (415 newborn babies every hour). The vast majority of neonatal deaths occur in South Asia and Sub Saharan Africa. Half of the 3.3 million neonatal deaths in 2009 were in five countries: India, Nigeria, Pakistan, China and Democratic Republic of Congo. Neonatal mortality constitutes 40percent of Under-5 Mortality and approximately 57percent of Infant Mortality (Black et al., 2010; WHO, 2011b).

Population / Indicator	World	High Income Countries	Low Income Countries
Population	6.9 Billion	1.24 Billion	5.66 Billion
Births per year	140 Million	14 Million	126 Million
Infant Deaths per year	6.38 million	80,133	6.3 Million
Neonatal deaths per year	3.6 million	45,700	3.4 million
Neonatal Deaths per day	9970	125	9845
Neonatal deaths per minute	7	0.11	6.89

Neonatal deaths calculated as 57% of Infant deaths
Source: Population Reference Bureau 2010

Table 1. Global Births and Neonatal Deaths 2010.

The global neonatal mortality rate ranges from as low as 1/1000 (e.g. Japan, Singapore) to as high as 53/1000 (e.g. Somalia, Afghanistan) (WHO, 2011). Among the WHO regions (Table 2), the African region has the highest average NMR (36/1000) and the European region the lowest average NMR (7/1000). The NMR ranges from 2-5 per one thousand live births in most European and other high income countries (Euro-Peristat, 2008). Although South East Asia has the second highest average NMR (31/1000), the highest absolute number of neonatal deaths occurs in this region because of population density. India alone contributes one quarter of global neonatal deaths. Combined, the African and South East Asian regions are sites of two thirds of global neonatal deaths (Lawn, 2005 & WHO, 2011). The global analyses of neonatal deaths are based on estimates because most neonatal deaths occur at home and are unrecorded in any formal registration system. Therefore, the global toll of neonatal deaths is probably much worse than what appears in published reports.

WHO Region	Regional NMR	Lowest NMR (Countries)	Median NMR (Countries)	Highest NMR (Countries)
African Region	36	7 (Seychelles) 9 (Mauritius)	39 (Nigeria) 42 (Angola)	51 (D R Congo) 50 (Mali)
South East Asia Region	31	8 (Thailand/Maldives) 9 (Sri Lanka)	19 (Indonesia) 18(Democratic People's Republic of Korea)	34 (India/Bhutan) 33 (Lesotho)
Eastern Mediterranean Region	30	4 (Qatar/ UAE) 6 (Bahrain)	20 (Morocco) 37 (Sudan)	53 (Afghanistan/Somalia) 42 (Pakistan)
Western Pacific Region	11	1 (Japan / Singapore) 3 (Australia)	11 (China) 15 (Philippines)	30 (Cambodia) 26 (Papua New Guinea)
Region of Americas	9	3 (Cuba) 4 (USA/Canada)	12 (Brazil/Colombia) 17 (Guatemala)	27 (Haiti) 23 (Trinidad and Tobago)
European Region	7	1 (Andorra/Iceland) 3 (UK/Austria)	12 (Turkey) 15 (Kazakhstan)	24 (Tajikistan) 20 (Turkmenistan)

Source: World Health statistics 2011, WHO

Table 2. Global Neonatal Mortality Rates 2011.

Over the last decade the neonatal deaths have gained an increasing importance on the world wide policy agenda because neonatal mortality now accounts for 41percent of Under 5 Childhood Mortality, which, according to WHO's millennium development goal (MDG) # 4 must be reduced by two thirds by 2015. Unfortunately, an equal number of babies die before birth. These still born babies are neither counted in the MDG's, nor in the Global Burden of Disease (GBD) metrics by WHO. Hence still births remain an invisible entity, though, during 2008, the estimated global number of still births was 2.65 million with an uncertainty range of 2.08 million to 3.79 million. (Lawn, J E. 2011). Although global neonatal mortality has improved significantly over the last two decades, the Perinatal mortality remains rather static, even in high income countries, because still birth rate has declined only by 14.5percent (from 22.1/1000 in 1995 to 18.9/1000 in 2009). (Cousens, S. 2011)

4. Neonatal mortality in low birth weight, preterm and non viable babies

The increasing survival of low birth weight and preterm babies over the last three decades has brought many challenges in estimating the true neonatal mortality and generating comparative analyses between countries and regions. Similar difficulties occur when babies are delivered at the limits of viability or born with lethal congenital anomalies. Various aspects of these issues are discussed in the following section.

4.1 Birth weight and neonatal mortality

The association between birth weight and mortality is among the strongest in epidemiology (Bosso, 2006). Although birth weight alone may not be the cause of mortality, the association is robust. Babies weighing less than 1,500g have a mortality risk at least 100-fold higher than babies at the optimum weight (the weight associated with the lowest mortality).Babies with a low birth weight are also at higher risk of long-term cognitive and motor impairments (Wilcox,

2001). Therefore birth weight is used as a very strong indicator to predict an individual baby's intact survival. The proportion of babies with a birth weight < 2500g is also used very widely as an indicator for assessing the population at risk, and historical series exist for many countries (Euro-Peristat, 2008). The relative risk (RR) of neonatal mortality decreases with increasing birth weight. According to PEARL Study's recent comparative analysis of birth weight specific neonatal mortality between the State of Qatar and Vermont Oxford Network (VON) expanded data base, the decline in RR is very sharp between birth weight categories 500g to 1500g (Table 3). As compared to babies with normal birth weight (≥ 2500g), the RR of mortality is 25 times, 17 times and 5.5 times higher (p <0.001) in babies with birth weight between 500- 750 g, 751-1000g and 1001-1500g respectively. In babies with birth weight > 1500g the RR is 1.5 times higher (p <0.001) (Salameh K, 2011).

Birth Weight (Grams)	Qatar 2010 n (%)	RR(95% CI) * *P*	VON 2007 n (%)	RR(95% CI)** *P*
501-750	15 (44.1)	24.7(13.5-45.4) <0.001	3938 (44.4)	25.1(23.6-27.4) <0.001
751-1000	15 (30)	16.8(8.9-31.7) <0.001	1668 (14.2)	7.9(7.4-8.8) <0.001
1001-1500	16 (9.8)	5.5(2.8-10.7) <0.001	1366 (4.9)	2.7(2.6-3.1) <0.001
1501-2000	7 (2.7)	1.5(0.6-3.6) 0.357	340 (2.5)	1.4(1.3-1.6) <0.001
2001-2500	9 (3)	1.7(1.1-5.5) 0.053	356 (2.2)	1.2(1.1-1.4) 0.001
≥2500	17 (1.7)	1	762 (1.7)	1

* Category wise (vertical) comparison of RR of Mortality Qatar 2010
** Category wise (vertical) comparison of RR of Mortality VON 2007

Table 3. The RR of mortality for each birth weight category as compared with normal birth weight (≥ 2500g) category:
State of Qatar (2010) and Vermont Oxford Network (2007) expanded data base.

4.2 Gestational age and neonatal mortality

Preterm deliveries are a major cause of neonatal deaths. Worldwide, prematurity and its complications constitute 12percent of global under five mortality and 30percent of neonatal mortality (Figs. 5). In absolute numbers, this makes approximately one million neonatal deaths per year. In high income countries, which have low neonatal mortality rates, prematurity is the biggest cause of neonatal mortality. In low income countries, which have high neonatal mortality rates, the proportion of deaths due to prematurity drops with increasing NMR. This fall is due to the large number of deaths from infections in high NMR countries. In a country with a very high NMR, the risk of death due to prematurity is still three times higher than a country with low NMR (Lawn et al., 2005). This is due to very limited resources and very high number of neonatal deaths in high NMR countries. The NMR is inversely proportional to the gestational age: the smaller the gestation age, the higher the mortality. PEARL Study's recent analysis (Rahman et al., 2011) has shown that the relative risk (RR) of death decreases significantly with increasing gestational age which is shown in Fig. 4A below.

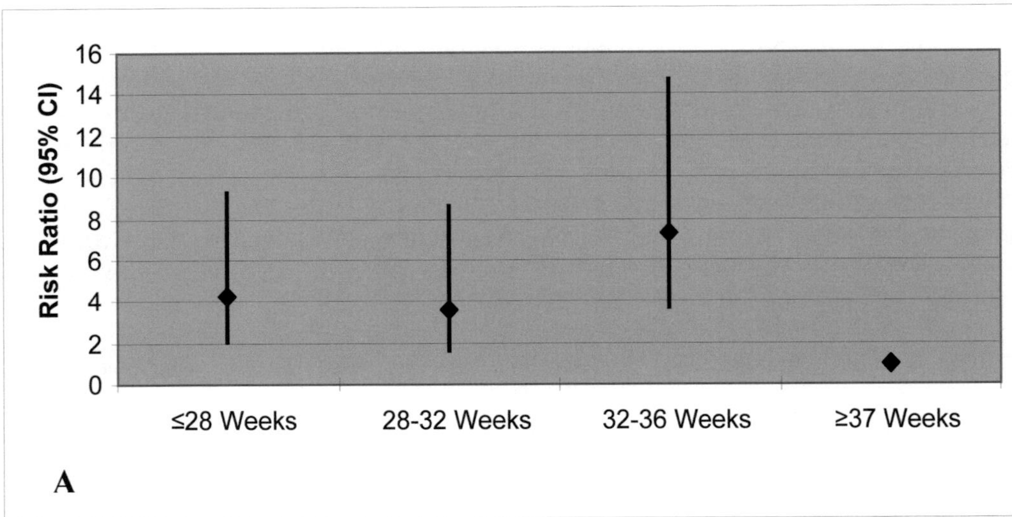

(Source: Rahman et al., 2011)

Fig. 4. A. Gestational Age wise Relative Risk of Neonatal Mortality
Relative risk calculated by taking immediate next category as reference.

When compared with babies born at term (Fig. 4B), the relative risk (RR) of mortality is 113.17, (95% CI 64.45-198.7;*P*<0.0001) among extremely preterm babies (≤ 28 weeks gestation), 26.4 (95% CI 11.91-58.55, *P*<0.0001) among very preterm babies (28^{+1}-32 weeks gestation) and 7.32 (95% CI 3.63-14.75; *P*<0.0001) among moderately preterm babies (32^{+1}-36^{+6} weeks).

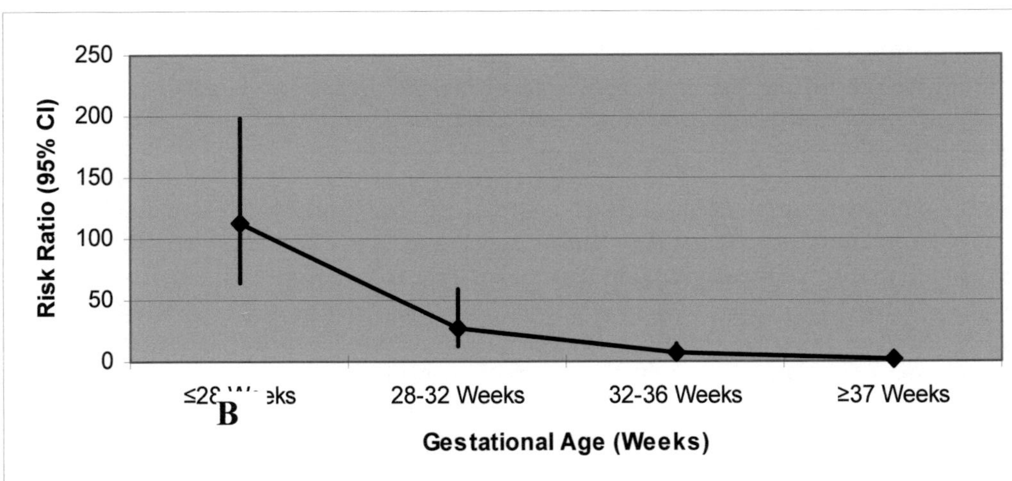

(Source: Rahman et al., 2011)

Fig. 4. B. Gestational Age wise Relative Risk of Neonatal Mortality Relative Risk calculated by taking Term babies (last category) as reference.

4.3 Adjusted neonatal mortality

For full term babies (≥ 37 weeks), the neonatal period extends from birth till 28th day of life. However, the exact duration of neonatal period for preterm babies is not well established. With the increasing survival of extremely preterm babies, it is becoming important to establish some rules to adjust for the duration of prematurity and calculate adjusted neonatal mortality rates. This will render the comparative analyses between neonatal units, countries and individual studies more homogenous. The exact estimate of gestational age at birth has always been a challenge both for obstetricians and neonatologists. Traditionally, the first day of maternal last menstrual period (LMP) has served as a basis for this estimation.

However, the accuracy of LMP can be doubtful in many cases. LMP combined with obstetric ultrasound during antenatal visits provide better estimates. However, antenatal care and the facility to undertake a reliable obstetric ultrasound may not always be available, particularly in disadvantaged localities/communities. A postnatal assessment of the baby by an experienced paediatrician using standard scoring test e.g. Ballard's Scoring System, can provide a better estimate in doubtful cases. In PEARL Study, we have used all three methods (LMP, Obstetric USS and Ballard's scoring system) to estimate the correct gestational age in doubtful cases (Rahman et al., 2011).

Gestation (Weeks)	Adjustment for Prematurity	+ Term Neonatal Period	Total Neonatal Period
24	90 days	+ 28 days	118 days
25	83 days	+ 28 days	111 days
26	76 days	+ 28 days	104 days
27	69 days	+ 28 days	97 days
28	62 days	+ 28 days	90 days
29	55 days	+ 28 days	83 days
30	48 days	+ 28 days	76 days
31	41 days	+ 28 days	69 days
32	34 days	+ 28 days	62 days
33	27 days	+ 28 days	55 days
34	20 days	+ 28 days	48 days
35	13 days	+ 28 days	41 days
36	6days	+ 28 days	34 days

Table 4. PEARL Study method of estimation of adjusted neonatal mortality.

In order to estimate the adjusted neonatal mortality for PEARL Study, we adopted the following rules. For all preterm babies, the neonatal period is extended in order to compensate for their prematurity. For example, a baby born at 24 completed weeks of gestation is born 90 days earlier before he/she would have been term (37 completed weeks of gestation). After becoming term (at 37 weeks), the baby's neonatal period will be counted, like any other term baby i.e. for another 28 days. This will make up a total of 118 days of neonatal period for a baby born at 24 completed weeks of gestation. During this extended neonatal period (118 days), the baby usually stays in neonatal intensive care unit (NICU). In case the baby dies during this period, his/her death is classified as neonatal death.

However, some extremely preterm babies stay in NICU longer than their adjusted neonatal period usually due to complications of prematurity and/or of intensive care procedures. In this case, their death after the adjusted neonatal period is classified as post neonatal death.

During the adjusted neonatal period, the first seven days will be considered as early neonatal period irrespective of the gestation at birth and the rest of the adjusted neonatal period as late neonatal period. Therefore, for an extremely preterm baby born at 24 weeks of gestation, the total neonatal period will be 118 days with first seven days counted as early neonatal period and the remaining 111 days counted as late neonatal period. Table 4 depicts a working table developed by The PEARL study in order to adjust the neonatal period for preterm babies born at various gestational ages, and to calculate their adjusted neonatal mortality rates for valid comparative analyses with other studies.

4.4 Limits of viability and neonatal mortality

The survival of preterm babies has improved exponentially over the last three decades resulting in gradual lowering of the limits of viability from 28 weeks to 24 weeks in 1990's, and most recently to 22 weeks (Euro-Peristat, 2008). However, the practice varies in individual countries and population groups. Evans and Levene (2001) reported that studies can exaggerate neonatal survival by 100percent at 23 weeks and 56percent at 24 weeks. This is a major issue in high income countries, which routinely provide care to extremely preterm babies born at the limits of viability. Therefore, while estimating and comparing neonatal mortality between countries, it is important to remove selection bias at the limits of viability. The WHO and UNICEF's annual neonatal mortality reports exclude babies <1000 grams and < 28 weeks gestation from each country's data to generate a reasonable comparison for low income countries, which do not provide care to extremely preterm and extremely low birth weight babies due to resource constraints (UNICEF, 2011).

4.5 Futility and neonatal mortality

Some babies are either very sick or extremely premature at birth or may be born with lethal congenital anomalies incompatible with life. These babies may not be resuscitated in labour room or provided intensive care because of futility. These neonatal deaths, which usually occur in labour and delivery suites, may not be reported in unit-based studies (Evans & Levene, 2001). Similarly legal frameworks, clinical guidelines and practice of termination of pregnancies varies widely between countries and cultural groups, which affects overall perinatal and neonatal mortality (Papiernik et al., 2008). These variations in policy and practice generate variations between populations of very preterm births among countries. In the MOSAIC Study cohort (Europe), pregnancy terminations constituted between 1 and 21.5percent of all very preterm births and between 4 and 53percent of stillbirths. Most terminations were due to congenital anomalies (Papiernik et al., 2008).

4.6 Corrected neonatal mortality

The neonatal mortality, calculated after excluding babies born alive at limits of viability or ones with extremely low birth weight (< 500g) or babies with lethal congenital anomalies, is called Corrected Neonatal Mortality (Lau et al., 1985). The reporting of corrected neonatal mortality makes inter country comparisons more rational (Euro-Peristat, 2008). The WHO and UNICEF exclude babies with a birth weight < 1000g and < 28 weeks gestation in their annual reports of global neonatal mortality rates (UNICEF, 2011).

5. Plurality and neonatal mortality

Twin and multiple births are associated with higher neonatal mortality and morbidity. A large population based study of twin births from United States and Australia (Scher, A.I. 2002) has shown that twins have an approximately five fold increased risk of foetal death, seven fold increased risk of neonatal death, and four fold increased risk of cerebral palsy (CP) as compared to singletons. However, at birth weight < 2500 g, twins generally did better than singletons, both with respect to mortality and CP rates. Second born twins and twins from same sex pairs were at increased risk of early death but not of CP. Twins from growth discordant pairs and twins whose co-twin died were at increased risk of both mortality and CP. The highest rates of CP were in surviving twins whose co twin was either born (4.7 percent), or died shortly after birth (6.3 percent) or had CP (11.8 percent). In the Euro-Peristat project (2008), multiples were four to eight times likely to die as compared to singletons (Fig. 5). Although the incidence of twin deliveries has increased with the introduction of assisted reproductive technology, perinatal mortality is about 40percent lower after assisted as compared with natural conception (Helmerhorst et al., 2004).

6. Socioeconomic correlates of neonatal mortality

Improvement in neonatal and perinatal survival comes as part of a package of development of human society, which is a multifaceted process involving social, economic, cultural, educational and health care development. PEARL Study, in its recent study (Rahman, S. 2010), has shown that reduction in poverty, increase in maternal education, and improved perinatal health care are associated with improved maternal, neonatal and perinatal survival. A number of other sociocultural factors e.g. ethnicity and consanguinity are also associated with increased neonatal mortality.

6.1 Poverty and neonatal mortality

Extreme poverty is the world's biggest killer and the greatest cause of ill health and suffering across the globe (Kevany, 1996). Infant mortality, a very strong outcome indicator of ill health, is most sensitive to poverty (Jahan, 2008). Hence, increased socioeconomic development is associated with a consistent decline in infant mortality (Rahman et al., 2010). A recent study from Netherlands (Agyemang, C. 2009) has shown that neighbourhood income and deprivation are related to Small for Gestational Age (SGA) birth (OR 1.32, 95% CI 1.04-1.68). Another recent study from Japan has reported increased risk of early spontaneous abortions among women who smoke (OR 2.39, 95% CI 1.26-4.25) and women who work outside their home (OR 1.65, 95% CI 1.17-2.35).

The global estimates show that the neonatal mortality is highest in low-income countries (Table 5,) and consistently declines with increasing regional income (WHO, 2011). During 2009, the average NMR in low-income countries (36/1000) was nine times higher than the average NMR in high-income countries (4/1000) and 1.5 times the global NMR (24/1000). During 1990-2009, the NMR decreased by 23.4percent in low-income countries, compared to 33.3percent in high-income countries and 27.3percent worldwide (WHO, 2011).

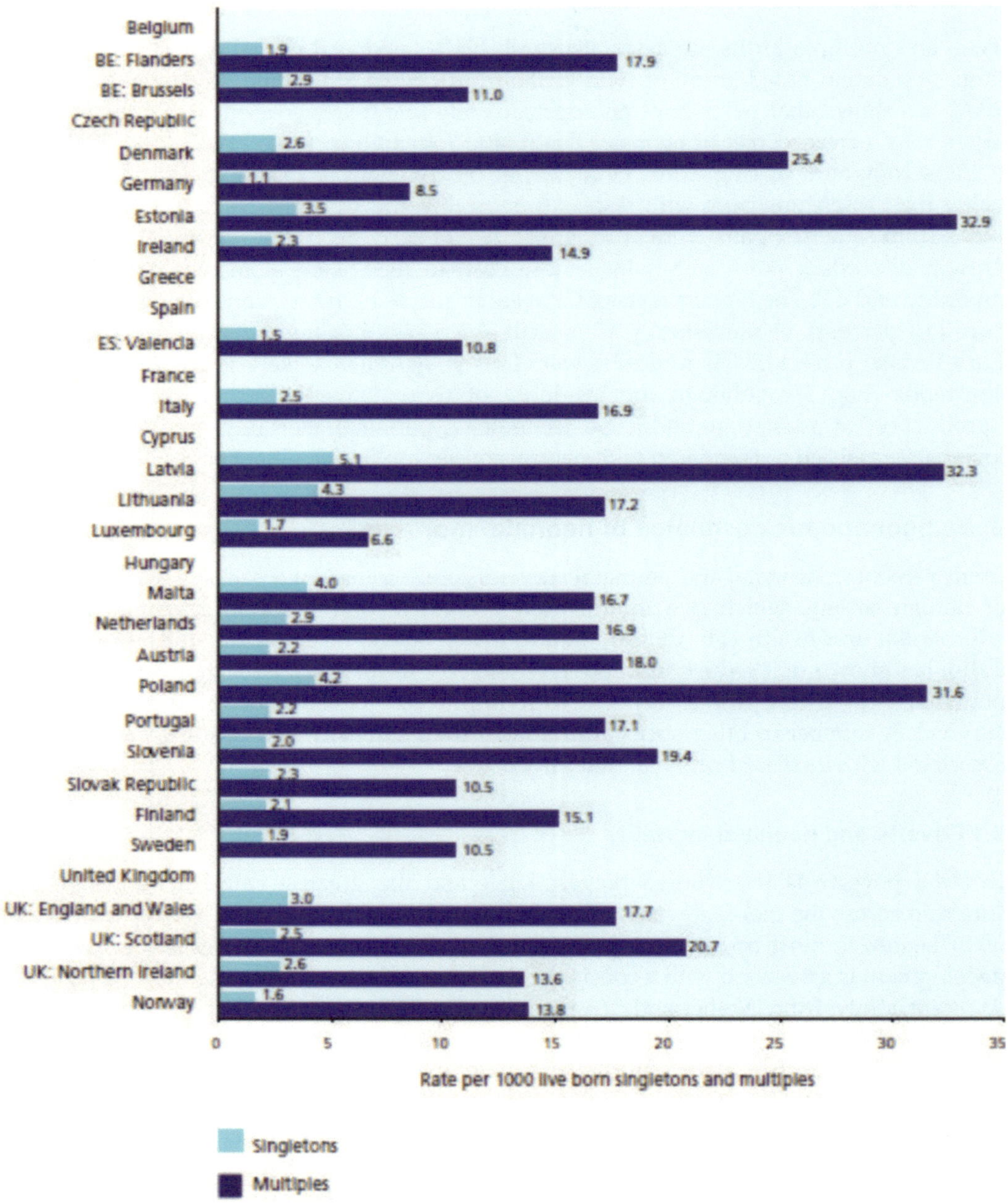

Fig. 5. Neonatal Mortality Rates (per 1000) in singleton and multiple births in Europe (Euro-Peristat, 2008).

Income Group	Neonatal Mortality Rate (per 1000 live births)		
	1990	2000	2009
Low Income	47	42	36
Lower Middle Income	36	32	26
Upper Middle Income	21	16	11
High Income	6	4	4
Global	33	29	24

Table 5. Neonatal Mortality by economic regions (WHO, 2011).

6.2 Maternal education and neonatal mortality

Maternal education is a very important socioeconomic indicator, which has known association with stillbirth, preterm births, low birth weight babies and neonatal and post neonatal mortality, which was confirmed by a ten years (1991-2000) population study based on birth certificate analysis from Quebec, Canada (Zhong-Cheng, L. 2006). The study also confirmed that the effects of maternal education were stronger than, and independent of, neighbourhood income (Fig. 6). Pregnant women with a low educational level have a nearly two fold higher risk of preterm birth than women with a high educational level (Jansen, P.W. 2009). The women with low educational attainment come from disadvantaged backgrounds with multiple adverse correlates. A recent study from Sweden (Sundquist, J. 2011) has shown that the Odds Ratio (OR) of giving birth to a Small for Gestation (SGA) infant for women living in high versus low deprivation neighbourhood was 0.38 (95% CI 1.32-1.44, $p<0.001$). Women with the highest risk of giving birth to an SGA infant were older; never married, widowed or divorced; had low family incomes; and/or the lowest educational attainment.

6.3 Ethnicity and neonatal mortality

The correlation between maternal ethnicity and neonatal mortality is variable. An Australian study (Ruan et al., 2011) found no influence of ethnicity on neonatal mortality (Caucasian, Asian, Indigenous and Polynesian Maori groups). However, ethnicity did influence foetal and neonatal growth and morbidity. Conversely, studies from multi ethnic European populations found an association between ethnicity and neonatal mortality. A study from Denmark (Villadsen et al., 2008), based on 23 years (1981-2003) data from a population registry (n = 1333452) described higher foetal and infant mortality among Turkish , Pakistani and Somali population as compared to the Danish population. The excess risk of mortality was not attributable to socioeconomic condition. A similar population based study from Brussels (Racape et al., 2010) reported increased perinatal mortality in particular ethnic groups, independent of socioeconomic status and maternal characteristics.

6.4 Consanguinity and neonatal mortality

Consanguinity has a known association with congenital anomalies, preterm births (Mumtaz G, 2010) and perinatal wastage (Assaf S, 2009). The global birth defects report by March of Dimes provides evidence to this. The Arab countries have the highest rates of birth defects. The same countries have the highest rates of consanguinity (40-70percent in general and up to 100percent in some tribes). With limited practice of antenatal terminations, these countries continue to have high neonatal and perinatal mortality rates (Salameh K 2009).

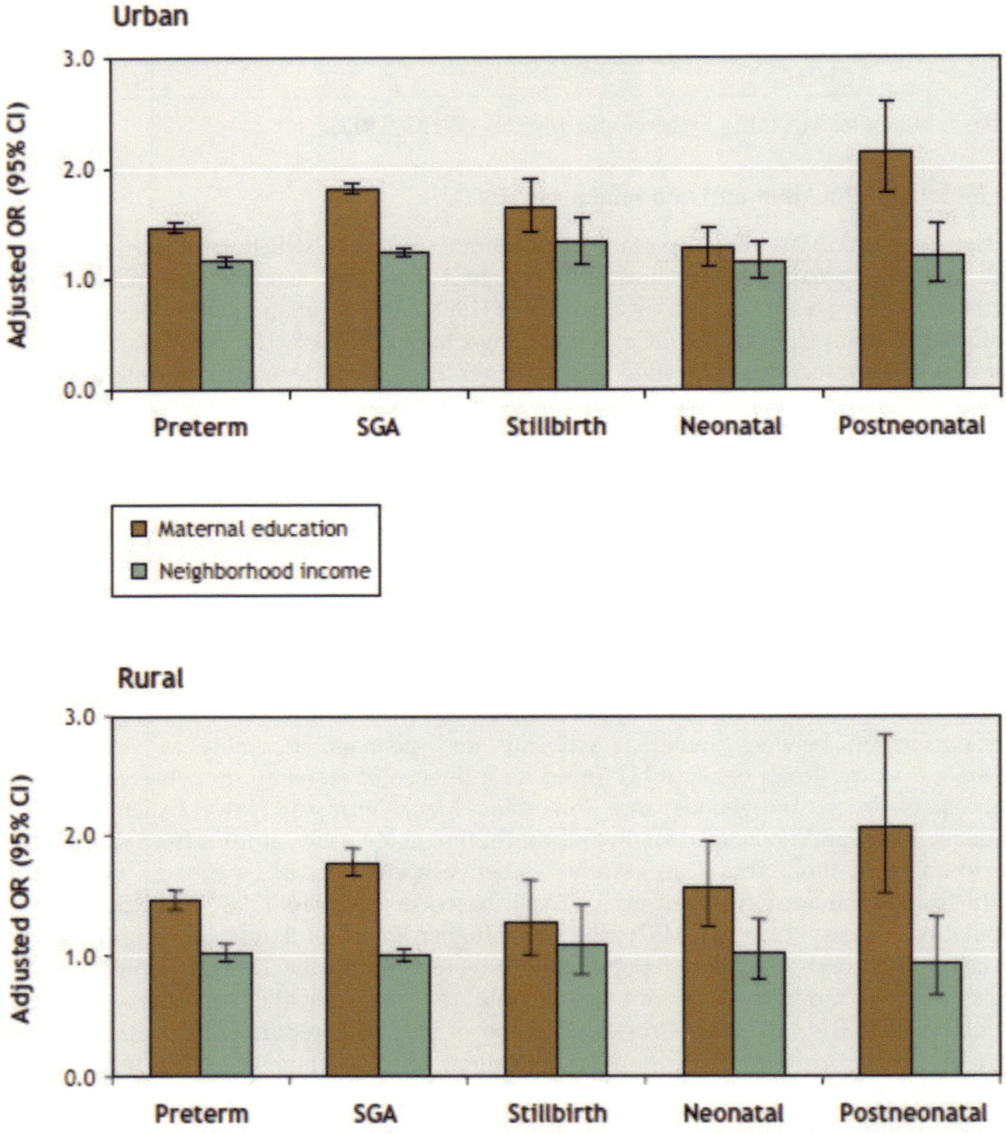

Source: (Zhong-Cheng, L. 2006)

Fig. 6. Adverse birth outcomes in Urban and Rural Quebec: A comparison of mothers not having graduated from high school with those having completed community college or some university, and mothers from poorest neighbourhood compared with mothers from richest neighbourhood.

7. Calculation and reporting of neonatal mortality

7.1 Period neonatal mortality and cohort neonatal mortality

Neonatal mortality is usually estimated as period mortality (all neonatal deaths per 1000 births during a specific period of time). In period mortality, the neonatal deaths include babies who were born immediately prior to the period but died as a neonate during the study period. On the other hand, the period mortality excludes those babies who were born at the end of the study period but died as neonate after the study period had ended. In general, the gain of deaths in the beginning of the study is balanced by the loss of deaths at the end of the study with little, if any, statistical difference. However, a true estimate of neonatal mortality can be done only by a cohort neonatal mortality, which includes only neonatal deaths per 1000 total births during a selected period. This necessitates the follow-up of the birth cohort until the end of the neonatal period of the last-born baby in the cohort.

This may take a few months in case of extremely preterm babies in which neonatal mortality needs adjustment for the time these preterm babies were born preterm. It is very important to report the exact definition of a given cohort during the publication of institution based neonatal mortality data. Some cohorts can be very selective e.g. cohorts which exclude babies < 500g at birth, or babies with lethal congenital anomalies or babies born alive but not resuscitated because of futility or non viability. Therefore, studies with very selective cohorts usually report significantly higher neonatal survival (Evans & Levene, 2001). This can be a significant problem at the limits of viability. Evans and Leven (2001), analyzed 67 studies (survival outcomes of 55 cohorts of < 28 weeks gestation babies) and estimated that the survival was exaggerated by 100percent at 23 weeks and 56percent at 24 weeks of gestation between the studies ($p<0.01$).

7.2 Adjusted and corrected neonatal mortality

The neonatal mortality is adjusted for prematurity and corrected for futility and lethal congenital anomalies for comparative purposes (see section 5.3 and 5.6 above for details).

8. Causes of neonatal mortality

The most recent global estimate of causes of child mortality (Black et al., 2010) suggested that 41percent of deaths in 2008 were due to neonatal deaths (Fig 7). The causes of neonatal mortality are divided into direct and indirect causes of mortality.

8.1 Direct causes of neonatal mortality

According to the global estimates by Black et al. (2010), the most important causes of neonatal mortality (Table 6) were complications of preterm birth (12percent, 1.033 million deaths), birth asphyxia (9percent, 0.814 million deaths), sepsis (6percent, 0.521 million deaths) and pneumonia (4percent, 0.386 million deaths). Despite a continuous increase in the population of children < 5 years, their mortality rate is declining. However, the decline in mortality is greater in children aged between 1-59 months than in neonates (0-27 days). Hence the proportion of neonatal deaths increased from 37percent in 2000-03 to 41percent in 2008. Thus, the main causes of neonatal death – preterm birth complications, birth asphyxia, sepsis and pneumonia - have become even more important. The distribution of causes of neonatal death varies by regions and countries, correlating with the degree of neonatal mortality (Fig. 8). In very high neonatal mortality settings, almost 50percent of deaths are due to severe infection, tetanus and diarrhoea. In low neonatal mortality settings, sepsis and pneumonia account for < 20percent of deaths, while tetanus and diarrhoea become almost non-existent as a cause of neonatal death.

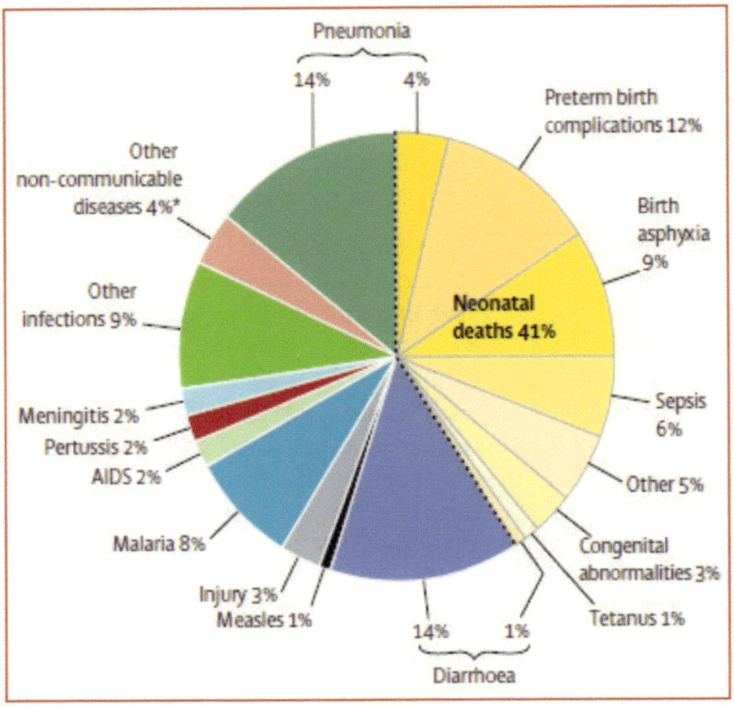

Fig. 7. Global Causes of Neonatal (0-27 days) and Child (1-59 months) Mortality, Source: (Black, 2010).

Cause of Neonatal Death (0-27 days)	Estimated Number (UR; millions)
Preterm birth complications	1.033 (0.717-1.216)
Birth asphyxia	0.814 (0.563-0.997)
Sepsis	0.521 (0.356-0.735)
Other	0.409 (0.318-0.883)
Pneumonia	0.386 (0.264-0.545)
Congenital abnormalities	0.272 (0.205-0.384)
Diarrhea	0.079 (0.057-0.211)
Tetanus	0.059 (0.032-0.083)
Total Global Neonatal Deaths	**3.573 million**

(UR: Uncertainty Range is defined as 2.5-97.5 centile) Source: (Black, 2010)

Table 6. Estimated global number of Neonatal deaths by cause 2008.

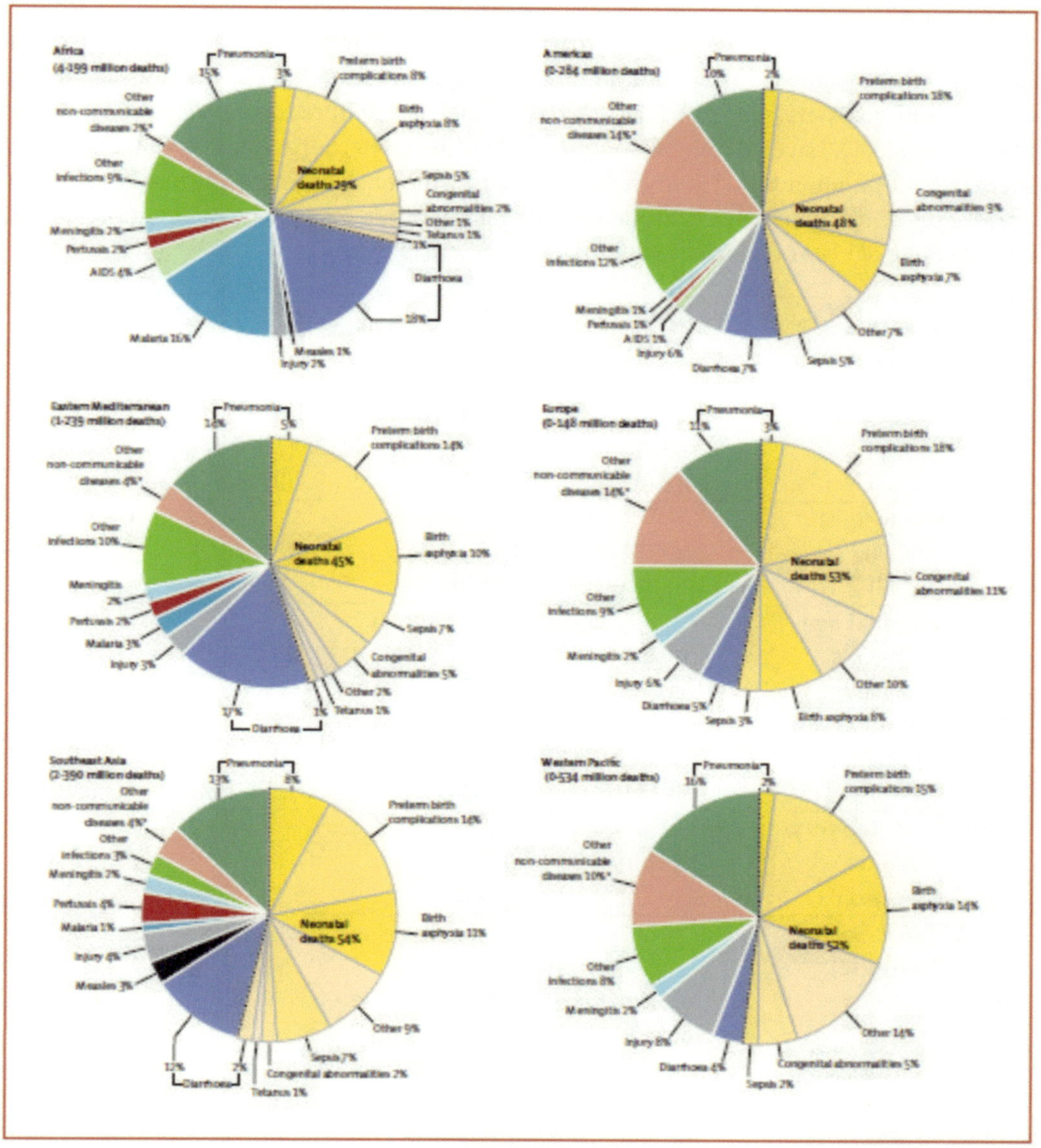

Source: (Black 2010)

Fig. 8. Regional Causes of Neonatal (0-27 days) and Child (1-59 months) Mortality.

The risk of neonatal death due to severe infections and asphyxia in very high neonatal mortality countries as compared to low neonatal mortality countries is about 11 and 8 fold respectively (Lawn et al., 2005). Although the proportion of deaths due to prematurity drops with increasing NMR, the risk of mortality due to prematurity is three times higher in high neonatal mortality countries as compared to low neonatal mortality countries (Lawn et al., 2005). The causes of neonatal death may also vary within the same country depending upon the socioeconomic status of the regional population and access to health care services.

8.2 Indirect causes of neonatal deaths

A number of indirect maternal and perinatal determinants affect neonatal outcomes. Maternal health before, during and after pregnancy, conditions at the time of labour and delivery and post natal care of babies play a significant role in reducing neonatal mortality. Jehan et al. (2009), have documented direct and indirect determinants of neonatal mortality in a recent population based study from Pakistan, which has the third highest NMR in the world. PEARL study has also documented similar determinants of neonatal mortality (Table 7) in the State of Qatar which has very low NMR (4/1000).

Variable	Dead N=44	Alive N=117	Odds Ratio (95%CI)	P- value
Fetal growth				
AGA	30(78.9)	91(78.4)	1 ref	0.028
SGA	7(18.4)	7(6.0)	3.0(1.1-9.4)	
LGA	1(2.6)	18(15.5)	0.2(0.1-1.3)	
Birth weight				
<2500g	32(72.7)	14(12.1)	19.4(8.2-46.2)	<0.001
≥2500 g	12(27.3)	102(87.9)	1 ref	
Gestational age				
<37 weeks	27(62.8)	12(10.3)	14.8(6.2-34.8)	<0.001
≥37 weeks	16(37.2)	105(89.7)	1 ref	
Presentation at birth				
Cephalic	29(82.9)	113(96.6)	1 ref	0.009
Breech	6(17.1)	4(3.4)	5.8(1.5-22.0)	
Mode of delivery				
Vaginal	24(54.5)	88(75.2)	1 ref	0.012
C-Section	20(45.5)	29(24.8)	2.5(1.2-5.2)	
APGAR Score (1 minute)				
≤6	26(61.9)	1(0.9)	*	<0.001
>6	16(38.1)	116(99.1)		
APGAR score (5 minutes)				
≤6	14(32.6)	0	*	<0.001
>6	29(67.4)	117(100)		
Delivery room resuscitation				
Yes	27(65.9)	7(6.0)	1 ref	<0.001
No	14(34.1)	110(94.0)	30.3(11.1-82.3)	

(Source: PEARL study Statistics 2011)
(* Valid odds ratio not calculated due to very few numbers in one category, ref=reference category, p value based on chi square or fisher exact test where the expected cell count is <5, odds ratio based on univariate logistic regression)

Table 7. Determinants of neonatal mortality, State of Qatar 2011.

9. Global trends in neonatal mortality (1970-2010)

Childhood mortality is a major concern for health care strategists, policy makers and planners. Although worldwide, the childhood mortality rates, including neonatal mortality rates, have declined since 1960s (Fig. 9, 10 & 11), the progress made has been alarmingly slow. This was recognized in the United Nation's Millennium Summit in 2000 which lead to the incorporation of Millennium Development Goal # 4 (MDG 4) in the World Millennium Declaration.

MDG 4 requires two thirds reduction in the deaths of children aged < 5 years by 2015. This required a reduction of childhood mortality at a rate of 4.4percent per year. According to a recently published review on reduction in neonatal, post neonatal, childhood and under five mortality by Rajaratnam et al. (2010); although significant progress has been made towards achieving MDG 4, many countries will fail to achieve the target by 2015. The two most recent annual World Health statistics published by WHO (2010 and 2011a) have also confirmed this fact.

From 1990 to 2010, the global rate of decline has been 2.1percent per year for neonatal mortality, 2.3percent for post neonatal mortality, and 2.2percent for childhood mortality against the required rate of 4.4percent per year. The under 5 mortality has been reduced from 16 million in 1970 to 11.9 million in 1990 to 7.7 million in 2010 which is more than 52% reduction in mortality over four decades (Fig. 9), despite an increase in total births by 16percent during the same period (Rajaratnam et al., 2010). Within the world regions, the reduction in under 5 mortality (all three components -- neonatal, post neonatal and childhood) is uneven (Fig. 10).

In 1970, South Asia and Sub Saharan Africa together accounted for 55 percent of all child mortality.

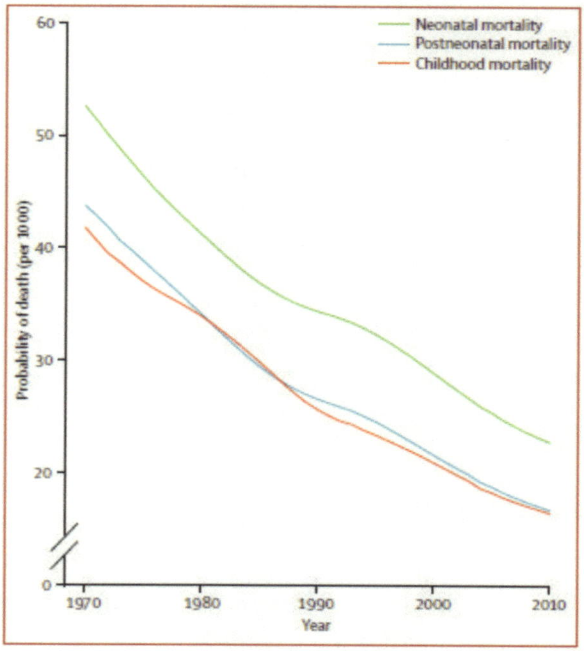

(Source: Rajaratnam et al., 2010)

Fig. 9. Worldwide neonatal, post neonatal and childhood mortality from 1970-2010.

In 2010, they accounted for more than 82percent (33percent in South Asia and 49.6percent in Sub Saharan Africa). The regions of Caribbean and Latin America, North Africa and Middle East, East and South East Asia have achieved 63percent reduction in child hood mortality between 1970 and 2010.

Some countries, e.g. the State of Qatar, have done exceptionally well by achieving all MDG's by 2007; just half way towards the target year 2015 (Qatar Statistics Authority, 2008). This is due to exceptional socio economic development and investment in perinatal health care in Qatar (Rahman et al., 2010).

Other countries (e.g. Sri Lanka, Nicaragua, Moldova, Indonesia, Honduras, Vietnam) have also done exceptionally well in reducing their neonatal mortality even though they have an annual GDP per capita < US $ 5000 (Martines et al., 2005). The improvement in Under 5 mortality has also been uneven between its three components. Most of the improvement has been in post neonatal (1-12 months) and childhood (1-5 years) mortality with slower progress in reducing neonatal mortality (Fig.9). Between 1970 and 2010, the global NMR decreased by 57percent (from 53/1000 in 1970 to 23/1000 in 2010); post neonatal mortality rate by 62percent and childhood mortality rate by 60percent. This decline resulted in neonatal mortality constituting 28 percent and 40 percent of Under 5 mortality in 2000 and 2010 respectively as opposed to 23percent in 1980. (Lawn et al., 2005; WHO, 2011a). Within the neonatal mortality, the decline in late neonatal mortality has been more significant than declines in early neonatal mortality (Fig. 11).

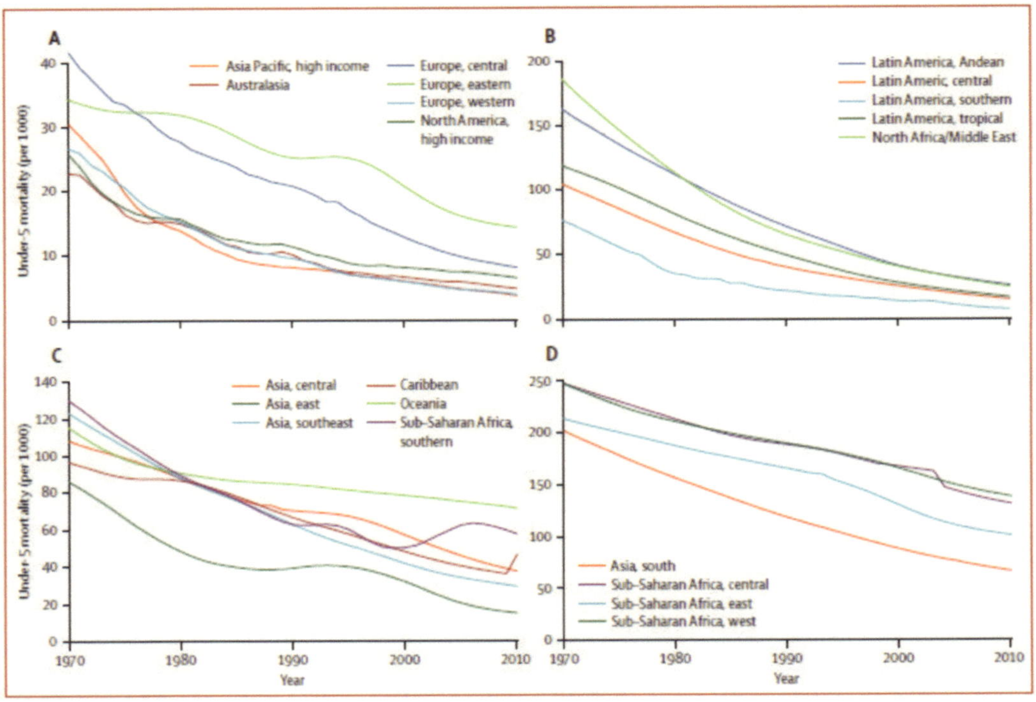

(Source: Rajaratnam, 2010)

Fig. 10. Regional neonatal, post neonatal and childhood mortality from 1970-2010.

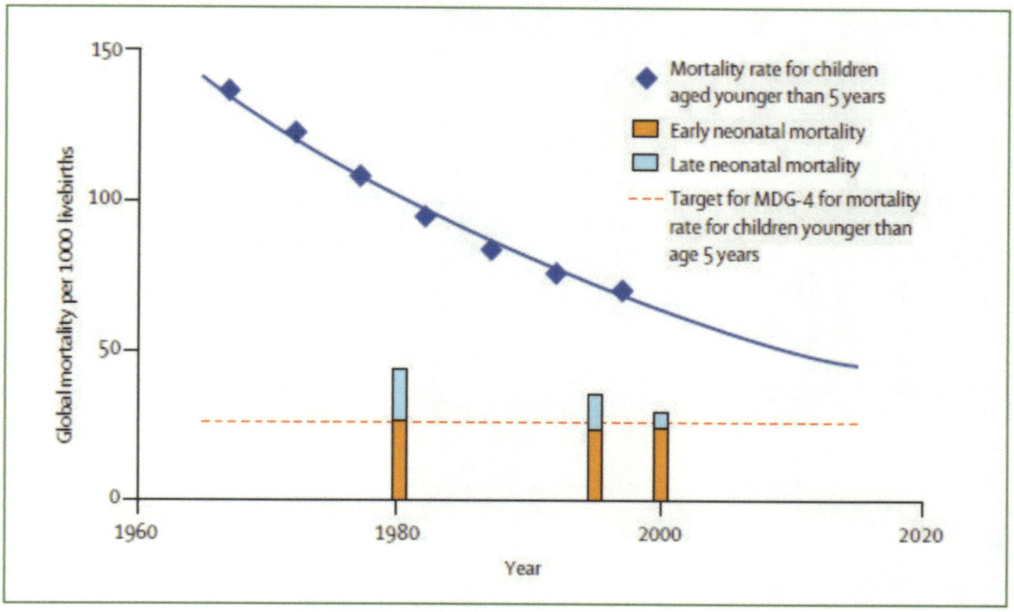

(Source: Lawn 2005)

Fig. 11. Meeting MDG-4: Trends in under 5 Mortality and Neonatal Mortality (Total, Early and Late) between 1965 & 2010.

10. Strategies to reduce neonatal mortality

Ever since the Millennium Declaration was announced, intense efforts began to achieve MDG's within the target period of 15 years (2000-2015). MDG-4 brought together individuals, organizations and media to draw comprehensive plans to ensure two thirds reduction in under 5 childhood mortality by 2015. Since 99 percent of childhood deaths occur in developing countries, which have constrained resources, the interventions must be cost effective, community based and within the reach of every citizen, particularly the urban, deprived and disadvantaged populations (The Lancet Neonatal Survival series, 2005). Significant progress has been made in reducing Under 5 childhood mortality over the last decade (2000-2010), though the progress towards reduction of neonatal deaths has been slow (Bhutta et al., 2010). A rapid progress is not only desirable; it remains a major challenge for the next five years (2011-2015).

Reduction of neonatal mortality is not a phenomenon in isolation. Improved neonatal survival should be seen as part of wider package (Fig 12) which should not only include care before, during and after pregnancy; it should also address wider issues of socioeconomic development including reduction in poverty and increased maternal education (Rahman 2010).

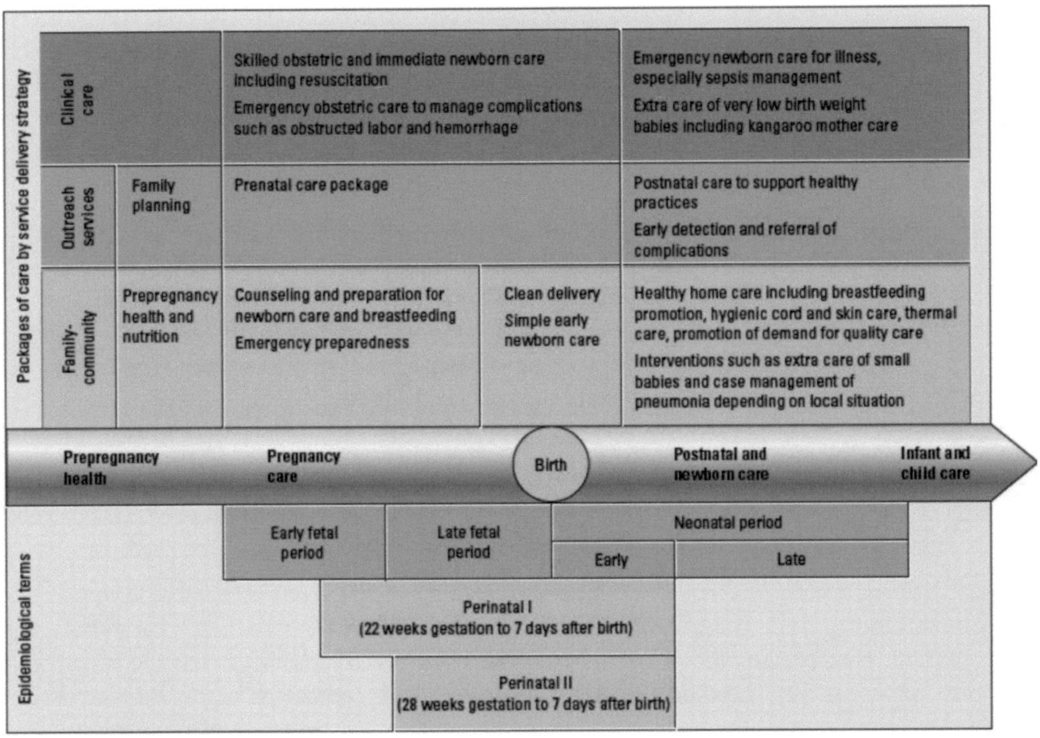

(Source: Lawn 2006)
Perinatal 1: for neonatal data collection as per International Classification of Diseases Version-10 (ICD-10);
Perinatal II: for international comparison of date as recommended by WHO

Fig. 12. The continuum of care for Mothers, Newborns and Children, showing epidemiological terms around the time of birth and packages of care relevant to Newborn health, according to service delivery level.

The Perinatal Health Care model developed by Lawn et al (2006) places neonatal mortality within the broad context of maternal and child health care. Strategies to reduce neonatal mortality should cover the whole continuum of care from maternal health before and during pregnancy to delivery, and early neonatal care to child health programmes (Fig. 12 middle bar). The model proposes three streams of service delivery strategies: clinical care, outreach services and family-community levels (Fig. 12 Upper part).

The clinical care strategies emphasize on provision of emergency and basic services in facilities and circumstances where minimum resources are available. The family planning strategies not only cater to prenatal health; they also take care of complications after delivery. Family-community level strategies include education and awareness of parents, families and public at large in health practices including clean delivery, breast feeding, basic newborn care and emergency preparedness. The model also highlights reporting of perinatal mortality for comparative analysis using WHO standards and alternative standards (Fig 12 Lower part). The model is extremely useful for low income countries which are struggling to reduce their very high burden of neonatal and perinatal mortality.

Looking at the whole picture of continuum of care, the first week of life is the most important period because 75percent of neonatal and 50percent of maternal deaths occur during this period. Maximum health coverage should be provided over these first seven days, particularly in disadvantaged and poor communities (Lawn et al., 2006). While the three direct causes of neonatal death (prematurity, asphyxia and sepsis) must be addressed, the indirect causes of neonatal deaths (low birth weight, poor maternal health, inadequate health care system, poverty and illiteracy) should also be addressed at all levels.

The State of Qatar is unique in having achieved all its MDG's by 2007 and hence provides an ideal model for study. The improved maternal, neonatal and perinatal survival in Qatar provides an example of how addressing wider community issues e.g. reduction in poverty, socioeconomic development, clean drinking water, sanitation, pest control, increased maternal education, investment in maternal and child health, high coverage antenatal and postnatal care, childhood vaccination and access to health care, can dramatically improve reproductive outcomes (Rahman 2010). Qatar's trends of maternal, neonatal and perinatal mortality since 1974 also provide an evidence that major reductions in mortality can be achieved through low cost community based interventions and not by high cost institutional investment. This gives a very strong message to low income countries that a lot can be achieved within their constrained resources.

10.1 Interventions to reduce neonatal mortality

Lawn and colleagues (2006) developed and categorized interventions to reduce neonatal mortality (Table 8), which addresses all periods of the continuum of care (pregnancy, intrapartum, postpartum and neonatal period). Some of these interventions are universally applicable because of their cost, feasibility and impact on mortality; others are more complex and are applicable only in relevant situations. This model led to the development of packages of intervention (Table 9) for universal scale up newborn care. These packages start from the family-community level and are carried over as essential, extra and emergency newborn care packages.

The Countdown to 2015 project (Bhutta et al., 2010) for maternal, newborn, and child survival monitors coverage of priority interventions to achieve MDG's for Child mortality and maternal health. The project has most recently reported on 26 key interventions in 68 countries, which account for more than 90percent burden of maternal and child mortality (Bhutta et al., 2010).

The median coverage of 20 interventions in 68 countries is shown in Fig. 13. According to this report, 19 countries were on track, 47 had accelerated and 12 countries showed decelerated progress in reducing childhood mortality. Progress towards reduction of neonatal mortality has been slow and maternal mortality remains high in most of these countries. However, there is strong evidence that rapid progress is possible. Focused and targeted interventions can reduce inequities related to socioeconomic status and gender. No country can afford not to seriously address neonatal care (Martinez et al., 2005).

Although NMR's are generally inversely correlated with GDP per capita; several low-income countries (e.g. Honduras, Indonesia, Moldova, Nicaragua, Sri Lanka, Vietnam) have achieved excellent reductions in their neonatal mortality rates (Fig. 14). Success is possible in low-income countries without the use of expensive high technology newborn care. The countries which have achieved excellent neonatal survival rates did so long before any expensive technology was introduced. In England, the NMR fell from more than 30/1000 in

1940 to 10/1000 in 1975, a reduction linked to the introduction of free antenatal care, improved care during labour, and availability of antibiotics (Mac Farlane et al., 1999). The State of Qatar achieved huge reduction in its NMR during the era of low cost, **community-based** interventions, backed by socioeconomic development (Rahman et al., 2010).

Period	Interventions for universal coverage (priority interventions for high-mortality settings)	Additional interventions (where the health care system has additional capacity and the NMR is lower; for example transition countries)	Situational interventions (where specific conditions are prevalent)
Prepregnancy	Family planning [B]:	Rubella immunization either of girls only or of all population if regular coverage can be maintained at more than 80 percent of the population [A]	HIV prevalent:
	• delay age of first pregnancy to after 18	Periconceptual or preconceptual provision of folate [A]	• primary prevention strategies [B]
	• space births by two to three years	Information counseling and support for	• voluntary counseling and testing and option of antiretroviral therapy [A]
	• provide opportunity to women to reduce births to their desired number and to avoid pregnancy after age 45	• smoking [RF A]	High prevalence of recessive conditions (such as sickle cell disease) or high rates of consanguineous marriages: offer genetics counseling [RF A]
	Prevention, identification, and management of sexually transmitted diseases [A]	• alcohol and drug abuse [RF A]	
	• iodination of salt [B]	• women experiencing violence [RF A]	
During pregnancy • Essential for all pregnancies	Four-visit prenatal care package, including • two tetanus immunizations [A]	Identification and treatment of bacteriuria [A] Information counseling and support for	HIV prevalent: primary prevention strategies [B]
	• iron and folate supplements [B]	• smoking cessation [RF A]	voluntary counseling and testing and option of antiretroviral therapy [A]
	• syphilis screening and treatment [A]	• alcohol and drug abuse [RF A]	
	• identification and referral of multiple pregnancy, abnormal lie, preeclampsia [B]	healthy diet and avoidance of unhelpful dietary taboos [C]	
	• birth planning and emergency preparedness [C]	women experiencing violence [RF A]	

Period	Interventions for universal coverage (priority interventions for high-mortality settings)	Additional interventions (where the health care system has additional capacity and the NMR is lower; for example transition countries)	Situational interventions (where specific conditions are prevalent)
	• prenatal counseling and preparation for breastfeeding [C]		
• Extra care for those at • risk of complications	Extra prenatal care (more frequent visits, more skilled caregiver) if • multiple pregnancy or abnormal lie (breech or transverse) [RF A] • pregnancy-induced hypertension or preeclampsia [RF A] • diabetes [RF A] • severe anemia [RF A] • previous fetal or neonatal death [RF A]	External cephalic version for breech presentation at 36 weeks [A] Fetal growth monitoring [A]	Malaria endemic : • intermittent presumptive treatment monthly after 20 weeks [A] • insecticide-treated bednets [B based on effect on LBW, not on NMR] Hookworm infestation prevalent: • presumptive treatment with mebendazole [B]
• Emergency for those with complications (first referral level and above)	Management of emergencies, including * preeclampsia or eclampsia [A] * bleeding in pregnancy [A *] * uterine infection [RF A]	In utero transfer of high-risk pregnancies [B]	Iodine deficiency prevalent: * iodine supplementation [B] Famine: * targeted food supplementation [B] Group B streptococcus prevalent: * screening and treatment [A]
Birth * Essential	Skilled care in labor, including * monitoring progress of labor (partograph), maternal and fetal well-being [A] * infection control [A *] **Newborn resuscitation** if required [A *}	Supportive companion in labor [A]	Mother HIV positive: • Antiretroviral therapy [A]

Period	Interventions for universal coverage (priority interventions for high-mortality settings)	Additional interventions (where the health care system has additional capacity and the NMR is lower; for example transition countries)	Situational interventions (where specific conditions are prevalent)
Extra care	Extra care if	Tocolytics in preterm labor and transfer to higher-level care if available [A]	Maternity waiting home if limited access to emergency obstetric care, high-risk condition identified, and culturally acceptable [B]
	• preterm (< 37 weeks) or prolonged (>18 hours) rupture of membranes or evidence of chorioamnionitis; give antibiotics to woman [A] • failure to progress in labor including instrumental vaginal delivery (vacuum) if required [RF A]	If preterm labor, then give prenatal steroid injection to mother [A]	
* Emergency	**Newborn resuscitation** if required [A*] Emergency obstetric care for acute intrapartum emergencies [A *] • obstructed labor and fetal distress • bleeding, infections, or eclampsia **Neonatal resuscitation** if required [A*]		
Postnatal and Newborn	Essential newborn care for all newborns, including	Trained breastfeeding counselors undertaking home visits [A]	Hepatitis B prevalent: Give hepatitis B immunization early [A]
Essential	early and exclusive breastfeeding [B]	Vitamin K (cost-effective as prophylaxis for all babies in transition countries) [B]	Mother HIV positive: provide counseling and support for feeding choices [C]
	warmth provision and avoidance of bathing during first 24 hours [C]	Routine newborn screening programs for sickle cell disease, glucose 6 phosphate dehydrogenase deficiency [B]	
	infection control including cord care and hygiene [B]		

Period	Interventions for universal coverage (priority interventions for high-mortality settings)	Additional interventions (where the health care system has additional capacity and the NMR is lower; for example transition countries)	Situational interventions (where specific conditions are prevalent)
	postpartum vitamin A provided to mother [B]		
	eye antimicrobial provided to prevent ophthalmia [A]		
	information and counseling for home care and emergency preparedness [C]		
Extra Care	Extra care for small babies (preterm or term IUGR) and multiple births, severe congenital abnormalities:	Provide special or intensive care for preterm babies [A]	Mother with tuberculosis: keep baby with mother and give isoniazid prophylaxis
	extra attention to warmth, feeding support, and early identification and management of complications [B]		Mother with syphilis: treat the baby even if symptomatic [A]
	kangaroo mother care [A: morbidity not mortality data]		
	vitmain K injection [B]		
Emergency	Emergency care providing specific and supportive care according to evidence-based guidelines for the following:	Provide special care for sick and small babies using skilled nurses and a higher nurse-to-patient ratio [B]	
	severe infections [A]		
	neonatal encephalopathy (following acute intrapartum insult)		
	severe jaundice or bleeding [A *]		
	neonatal tetatnus		

Note: A = rigorous meta-analysis or at least one good randomized controlled trial exists, RF A = evidence regarding risk is strong, B = well conducted clinical studies exist but no randomized controlled trial done, C = some descriptive evidence and expert committee consensus exists A*= unethical to test rigorously and widely practiced as standard (for example, blood transfusion, neonatal resuscitation). **Bold** text signifies priority packages or interventions considered in detail in this chapter.
Source: Authors, based on extensive literature review. References detailed on http://www.fic.nih.gov/dcpp/

Table 8. Interventions to Reduce Fetal and Neonatal Mortality by timing of intervention and by Scalability of Intervention.

Intervention package	Contents	Number of target population per year (millions)	Implementation Strategy	Estimated current coverage (percent) South Asia	Sub Saharan Africa	Reduction in all-cause NMR (percent)	Comments on evidence
Family-community care of the newborn at home after birth	Healthy home care practices (Exclusive breastfeeding, warmth protection, clean cord care, care seeking for emergencies); if birth outside a facility, then clean delivery kit	All newborn infants: World 130 South Asia and Sub-Saharan Africa 63	Women's groups and community health workers doing postnatal visits, with links to the formal health care system, including support for referral. If appropriate, extra care of moderately small babies at home and community-based management of acute respiratory infections.	36	28	10--40	Mortality reduction based on studies in high NMR settings with weak health systems. Extra care of LBW infants and community management of acute respiratory infections not included in range shown.
Essential newborn care at the time of birth	Immediate drying, warmth, early breast-feeding, hygiene maintenance, and infection prevention	All newborn infants: World 130 South Asia and Sub-Saharan Africa 63	Skilled attendant, or if no skilled attendant available, some simple postnatal practices are feasible at home with other cadres of workers	11	14	20 - 30	Based on conservative combining of single interventions (for example, breastfeeding) in the package
Neonatal resuscitation	Resuscitation after birth if required	Newborns not breathing at birth: World 6.5 South Asia and Sub-Saharan Africa 3.2	Skilled attendant	3	3	10 --25	Limited studies, mainly from lower NMR settings with high percentage of asphyxia deaths, so range from studies was reduced
Extra care of small new borns	Extra support for warmth (kangaroo mother care), feeding, and illness identification and management	LBW neonates: World 20.0 South Asia and Sub-Saharan Africa 10.7	Facility-based care for severely preterm babies: Community-based care is effective for moderately preterm babies	< 10	< 10	20- 40	Most studies are nonrandomized controlled trials at the community level in settings with extremely high LBW rates. Effect depends on baseline NMR and LBW rates
Emergency care of ill newborns	Management of ill infants, especially those with neonatal infections	Neonates with illnesses: World 13.0 South Asia and Sub-Saharan Africa 6.3	Facility-based care with antibiotics and supportive care. Community-based management with oral antibiotics for acute respiratory infections	< 20	< 20	20 - 50	Meta-analysis of effect on the NMR of oral antibiotic management of acute respiratory infections in the community in high-mortality settings

Intervention package	Contents	Number of target population per year (millions)	Implementation Strategy	Estimated current coverage (percent)		Reduction in all-cause NMR (percent)	Comments on evidence
				South Asia	Sub Saharan Africa		
Neonatal packages plus MCH package	Neonatal packages as above, in addition to family planning, prenatal care, and comprehensi ve obstetric car packages	All newborn infants: World 130 South Asia and Sub-Saharan Africa 63	Supply of care throughout pregnancy, childbirth and postnatal period with increased demand and improved referral systems	< 5	< 5	--	No study data identified. Marginal budgeting for bottlenecks tool suggests 58 percent in South Asia and 71 percent in Sub-Saharan Africa

Source: Local data or Darmstadt and other 2005: Knippenberg and others 2005; Lawn Cousens, and Zupan 2005

Note: The range of reduction of all-cause NMRs given for each package is independent of the others; hence the total is greater than 100 percent.

Table 9. Packages for Universal Scale-up of Newborn Care.

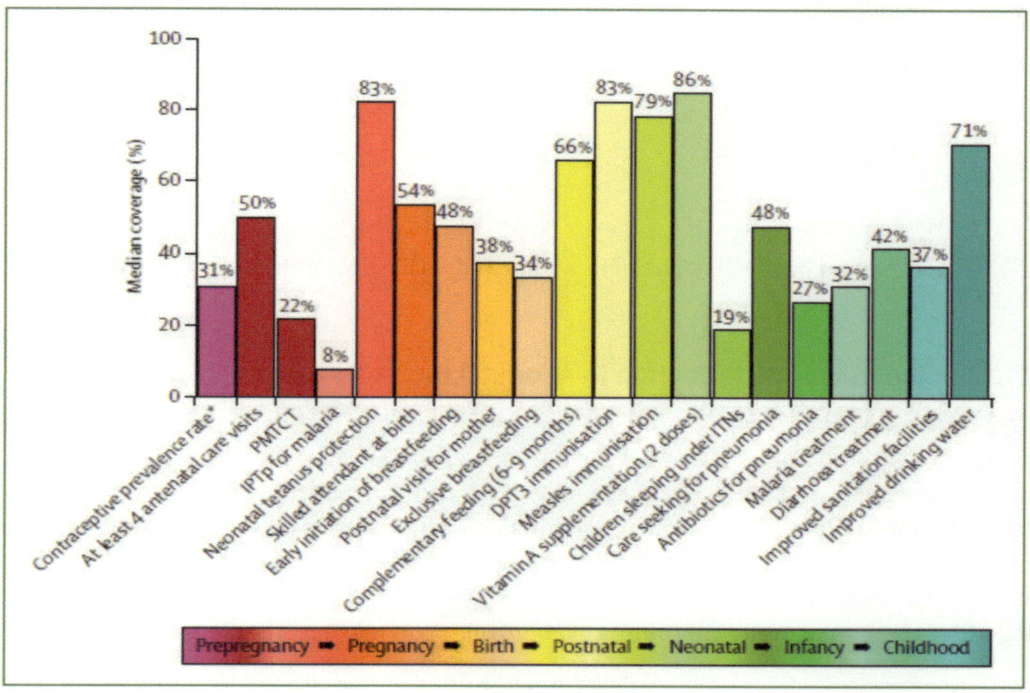

Source: (Bhutta et al., 2010)

Fig. 13. Median coverage for effective maternal, newborn and child interventions in 68 countries accounting for more than 90% of maternal and child deaths worldwide.

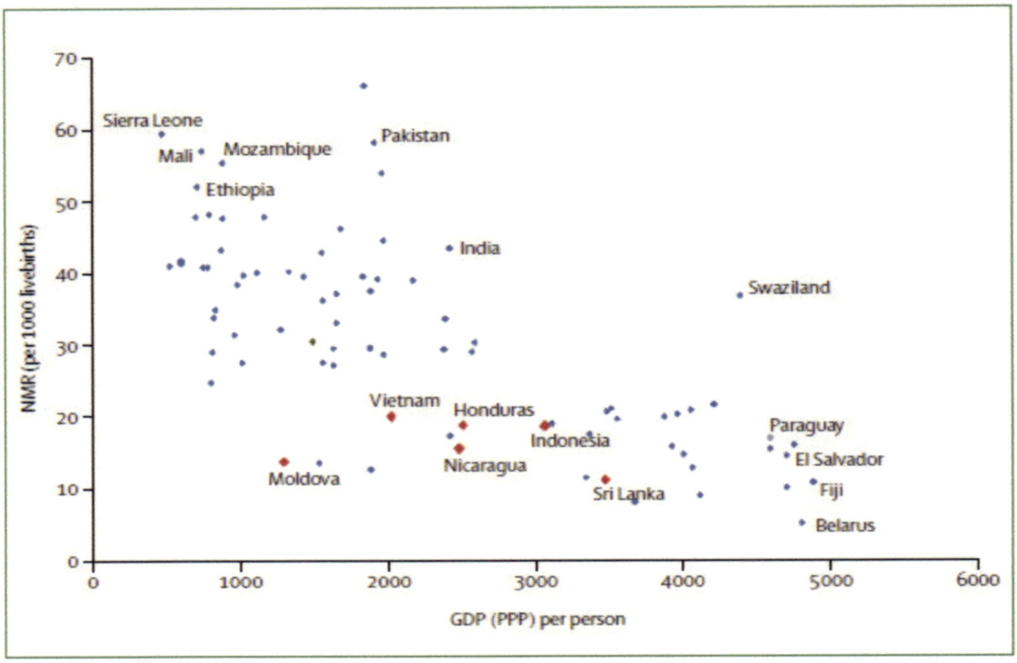

(Source: Martines, et al., 2005)

Fig. 14. Correlation between neonatal mortality and GDP per Capita < USD 5000 (in year 2000).

11. Challenges to the reduction in neonatal mortality and the way forward

Reduction of neonatal mortality has become the most significant challenge as the world progresses in its fight to reduce Under 5 childhood mortality. Socioeconomic and developmental in-equalities combined with low political priority of maternal and child health in most parts of the world, remain significant contributors of neonatal mortality. Poverty, illiteracy and lack of public awareness further intensify the grave situation. These wide spectrum challenges require a unified approach by the governments, public as well as the international organizations (Bhutta et al., 2010).

12. Case studies

Sri Lanka, Brazil and The State of Qatar are presented in separate panels as stories of success. These countries are excellent case studies in reducing neonatal mortality rates and achieving MDG 4 in resource constrained environment.

Sri Lanka – Achievement of excellent NMR using community based primary health care services

Sri Lanka had a population of 20 million with a GDP(PPP) per person of US $3470 in year 2000 when the NMR had already fallen to 10/1000. During this time, more than 6.6percent of the population was living on an income of < US$1 a day. Public expenditure on education and health was 1.3 percent and 1.8percent of GDP, respectively. The female literacy rate was high at 90percent. The first neonatal intensive care unit opened in mid-1980s in Colombo when the NMR was already < 20. In 1999, there were just 40 incubators and five neonatal intensive care units in the country. The great decline in neonatal mortality shown was not due, therefore, to the availability of high technology facilities, but was the result of sustained inputs into and use of primary care services and facilities in the government sector. Starting in 1913, health services for rural communities started receiving special attention in Sri Lanka. Midwives were posted to the rural areas to provide both home and institutional care. By 1996, there was one midwife for a population of 3000-5000. Outreach antenatal care is provided by these midwives, with antenatal coverage of almost 100percent in 1999. In 1996, 86percent of deliveries were in government hospitals, where a cadre of 2500 skilled hospital midwives attend services free of charge. There is also equitable and easy access to health care facilities throughout Sri Lanka. The average distance from every house to a health facility is 1.4 km, and from smaller hospital to the more advanced hospitals is only about 5 km. Government health facilities are used by both the poor and the rich, and efforts have been made to maintain high quality of service. (Source: Martinez et al., 2005)

Brazil – Moving from a high mortality country to achieving MDG's beyond targets

Brazil is a high mortality country that is on target to achieve MDG-4. In children < 5 years old, mortality has been dropping by about 5percent a year since 1990, which is substantially faster than the 4.4percent yearly reduction needed to reach the MDG target. Currently, 22 of every 1000 children die before their fifth birthday. The prevalence of underweight children < 5 years dropped from 5.7 percent in 1990, to 1.7 percent in 2006, and stunting fell from 19.9percent to 7.1percent in the same period. Overall progress has been accompanied by a sharp reduction in inequalities between socioeconomic quintiles. In 1996, about 30percent of all births to mothers in the poorest quintile did not receive skilled care, but by 2007, coverage was universal. Likewise, stunting prevalence fell from 40percent to 10percent in children in the poorest quintile between 1989 and 2007, remaining stable at around 3-5 percent in the richest quintile. These examples are only two of many indications of reproductive, maternal, newborn, and child health for which equity has improved in the past two decades.

Brazil's successful reduction of inequities cannot be attributed solely to one factor. Although economic growth has been moderate since 1990, income distribution has improved strikingly in recent years. A nationwide tax-based Unified Health System without any user fees was launched in 1989, and geographical targeting has guided deployment of family health teams of doctors, nurses, and community health workers in the poorest areas of the country. As a result, primary health-care coverage e.g. by skilled birth attendants, is now almost universal. Additionally, conditional cash transfer programmes cover about a third of the population, and several health sector initiatives-including immunization, HIV/AIDS control, and breast feeding promotion activities-have been highly successful. Perhaps more than any one policy or initiative, the reduction of regional and socio economic disparities in health and development has been a central element in Brazil's political agenda for the past 20 years, and this approach is now starting to bear fruit. (Source: Bhutta et al., 2009)

The State of Qatar – An exceptional example of achieving all MDG's by 2007

The State of Qatar stands unique among the world countries by having achieved all MDG's by 2007. The State provides universal access to health care including Maternal and Child Health care. A shift from home to hospital deliveries took place during 1970's. Since 1980, Qatar has achieved almost 100% coverage of its pregnancies and deliveries by trained birth attendants. Since 1974 a trained person has seen almost 100% of the newborn babies. The level of childhood immunization, which was 80% in 1980, reached 96-100% by 1986. The state had only three cases of neonatal tetanus in 1980 and one case in 1986. Since then there has been no recorded case of neonatal tetanus in Qatar. The Maternal Mortality Ratio (MMR) remained zero in 1993, 1995 and then from 1998 until 2000. For the rest of the years, MMR has been approximately 10/100,000. The major decline in Qatar's neonatal and perinatal mortality took place during the 1970's. By 1976 Qatar's NMR was 12/1000 and PMR 20/1000, both achieved by using very basic low cost neonatal technology (neonatal resuscitation, temperature control using incubators, infection control, fluid balance, breast feeding and care of low birth weight babies). Between 1974 and 1993 Qatar's overall per capita health expenditure increased only by 19%. During 1993-2008 Qatar's per capita health expenditure increased by 137%. This was the era of using very expensive high-tech neonatal intensive care, which resulted in the decline of NMR from 8.3 to 4.4.

Qatar's remarkable achievement of maternal, neonatal and perinatal survival was not a phenomenon in isolation. It has evolved as a part of the global socioeconomic and cultural changes in the society; the most important being reduction in poverty and increase in female literacy. Poverty, measured by the ratio of those with an income of < US$1 a day, has long been eliminated in Qatar. The state has a high rate as well as a high level of Female literacy (> 99%). Qatar's standard of living is very high with abundant across the board supply of clean drinking water, efficient sewerage, drainage, pest control, environmental control, public health awareness programs, communication, electricity and transportation facilities. The state of Qatar is a very good model to illustrate the fact that Neonatal Perinatal Survival is part of a package of development of human society which is a multifaceted process involving social, economic, cultural, educational and health care development. (Source: Rahman et al., 2010)

13. Conclusions

Although significant progress has been made in reducing childhood mortality over the last four decades; the progress in achieving targeted reduction in neonatal mortality remains very slow. The evidence shows that the targets are achievable with the use of packages of simple, cost effective and feasible interventions without the use of very high and expensive technology. Over the remaining one third period to achieve MDG 4 (2011-2015), newborn care must be placed on top priority, without which any further significant reduction in childhood mortality will remain a dream.

Funding: Perinatal Neonatal Outcomes Research Study in the Arabian Gulf (PEARL Study) has been funded exclusively by Qatar National Research Fund (QNRF) for a period of three years (December 2010 -Novembetr 2013), through its 3rd cycle of National Priorities Research Programme (NPRP). Grant # NPRP 09-390-3-097

Ethical Approval: PEARL study is approved by the Institutional Research Ethics Committee of Hamad Medical Corporation State of Qatar (protocol #9211/09).

Conflict of interest: None declared.

14. Acknowledgments

We thank *The Lancet* for permission to reproduce tables, graphs and figures from its series of publication on neonatal survival. We are also thankful to the authors of these articles, Robert Black, Joy Lawn, Zulfiqar Bhutta and their colleagues, for granting us permission to reproduce tables and figures. Our gratitude goes to Jennifer Zeitlin (INSERM France) for granting permission to use graphs from Euro-Peristat project report 2008.

We thank the PEARL study team for their support in data collection, analysis, interpretation and literature search; particularly Dr. Nuha Nimeri (Research Fellow); Dr. Sarrah El Tiniye (Research Associate); Dr. Emirah Tamano, Rabia Aman, Dr. Faiza Rani, Dr. Yasmeen Hamdi, Dr. Naseeba Muhammad, Dr. Saima Khan, Dr. Arjumand Afzal (Research Assistants); and Mohammad Tahir Yousafzai (Statistician). We are thankful to Dr. Hiba Tohid for her help in proof reading the manuscript.

We are thankful to Qatar National Research Fund (QNRF) for funding PEARL Study and the Medical Research Center, Hamad Medical Corporation for granting ethical approval and administrative support to PEARL Study.

15. References

Agyemang,C., Vrijkotte, T.G.M., Droomers, M., van der Wal, M.F., Bonsel, G.J., Stronks, K. (2009). The effect of neighbourhood income and deprivation on pregnancy outcomes in Amsterdam, The Netherlands. *J Epidemiol Community Health,* Vol. 63, pp. 755-60.

Assaf, S., Khawaja, M., DeJong, J., Mahfoud, Z., Yunis, K. (2009). Consanguinity and reproductive wastage in the Palestinian territories. *Pediatr Perinat Epidemiol,* Vol.23,pp.107-115

Australian Bureau of Statistics (2009). Perinatal Deaths, Australia. (www.abs.gov.au/AUSSTATS/)

Bhutta, Z.A., Chopra, M., Axelson, H., Berman, P., Boerma, T., Bryce, J……Wardlaw, T. (2010). Countdown to 2015 decade report (2000-10): taking stock of maternal, newborn, and child survival. *Lancet,* Vol. 375, No.9730, pp. 2032-44.

Black, R.E., Cousen, S., Johnson, H.L., Lawn, J.E., Rudon, I., Bassani, D.G…..Mather, C. (2010). Global, regional, and national causes of child mortality in 2008: a systematic analysis. *Lancet,* Vol. 375, No. 9730, pp. 1969-1987.

Basso, O., Wilcox, A.J., Weinberg, C.R. (2006). Birth Weight and Mortality: Causality or Confounding? *Am J Epidemiol.,* Vol. 164, pp. 303–311.

Cousens, S., Blencowe, H., Stanton, C., Chou, D., Ahmed, S., Steinhardt, L., Creanga, A.A., Tuncalp, O., Balsara, Z.P., Gupta, S., Say, L., Lawn, J.E. (2011). National, regional and worldwide estimates of still birth rates in 2009 with trends since 1995: a systematic analysis. *Lancet.*Vol,377.No,9774.pp,1390-30.

Evans, J.D., Levene, L.I. (2001) Evidence of selection bias in preterm survival studies: a systematic review. *Arch Dis Child Fetal Neontal Ed,* Vol. 84, No. 2, pp. F79-F84.

Euro-Peristat Project. 2008. European Perinatal Health Report (www.europeristat.com)

Helmerhorst, F.M., Perquin, D.A.M., Donker, D., Keirse, M. J. N. C. (2004). Perinatal outcome of singletons and twins after assisted conception: a systematic review of controlled studies.*BMJ,* Vol. 328,No. 7434, pp.261-5.

Jahan, S. (2008). Poverty and Infant Mortality in the Eastern Mediterranean region: a meta-analysis. *J Epidemiol Community Health,*Vol. 62, pp.745-51.

Jansen, P.W., Tiemeier, H., Jaddoe, V.W.V., Hofman, A., Steegers, E.A.P., Verhulst, F.C., Mackenbach, J.P. Raat. H. (2009). Explaining Educational inequalities in preterm birth: the generation r study. Arch Dis Child. Fetal Neonatal Ed. Vol, 94. Pp. F28-34.

Jehan, I., Harris, H., Salat, S., Zeb, A., Mobeen, N., Pasha, O.......Goldenberg, R.L. (2009). Neonatal mortality, risk factors and causes: a prospective population based cohort study in urban Pakistan. *Bull WHO*, Vol. 87, pp 130-138.

Kevany J. (1996). Extreme poverty: an obligation ignored. *BMJ*, Vol. 313, No. 1996, pp. 65-66.

Lack, N., Zeitlin, J., Krebs, L., Kunzel, W., Alexander, S. (2003). Methodological difficulties in the comparison of indicators of perinatal health across Europe. *Europ J Obstet Gynaecol Rep Biolo,* Vol. 111, pp. S33-S44.

Lawn, J.E., Cousens, S., Zupan, J. (2005). Four million neonatal deaths: When? Where? Why? *Lancet* (Neonatal Survival Series). Vol.365, No.9462, pp. 891-900.

Lawn, J E., Zupan, J., Begkoyian, G., Knippenberg, R. (2006). Neonatal Survival. Chapter 27 in Disease Control Priorities in developing countries. Second Ed. Oxford University Press & World Bank. Available from (http://www.dcp2.org/pubs/DCP) Accessed September 17th, 2011.

Lawn, J.E., Blencowe, H., Pattinson, R., Cousens, S., Kumar, R., Ibiebele, I., Gardosi, J., Day, L.T., Stanton, T., for the Lancet's Stillbirth steering committee. (2011). Stillbirths: Where? When? Why? How to make the data count? *Lancet,* Vol.377, pp. 1448-63.

Lau, S.P., Davies, D.P., Fung, K.P., Fok, T.F.(1985) Perinatal and neonatal Mortality in Hong Kong: An Appraisal. *Journal of Hong Kong Medical Association,* Vol. 37, No. 3, pp. 112-16.

Mac Farlane, A. J., Johnson, A., Mugford, M. (1999). Epidemiology. In Rennie J.M. Roberton, N.R.C. Eds. Textbook of Neonatology (3rd Ed). Edinburgh: Churchill Livingston. 1999: 3-33.Martines, J., Paul, V. K., Bhutta, Z. A., Koblinsky, M., Soucat, A., Walker, N..... Costello A. (2005). Neonatal survival: a call for action. *Lancet*, Vol. 365, pp. 1189-97.

Papiernik, E., Zeitlin, J. Delmas, D., Draper, E.S., Gadzinowski, J., Kunzel, W....Breat, G. (2008). Termination of Pregnancy among very preterm births and its impact on very preterm mortality: results from ten European population based cohorts in the MOSAIC study. *BJOG*, Vol. 115, pp. 361-368.

Population Reference Bureau. (2010). World Population data sheet. 2010. pp.1-19. (www.prb.org)

Qatar Statistics Authority. 2008. The Millennium development goals in the State of Qatar (2008). Available from (http://www.qsa.gov.qa). Accessed September 15th 2011.

Rahman, S., Salameh, K., Al-Rifai H., Masoud, A., Lutfi, S., Salama, H..... Bener, A. (2011). Gestational Age Specific Neonatal Survival in the State of Qatar (2003-2008) – A Comparative Study with International Benchmarks. JCPSP, Vol. 21, No. 9, pp.542-547.

Rahman, S., Salameh, K., Bener, A. El Ansari, W. (2010). Socioeconomic associations of improved maternal, neonatal, and perinatal survival in Qatar. *International Journal of Women's Health*, Vol. 2, pp. 311–318.

Rajaratnam, J.K., Marcus, J.R., Flaxman, A.D., Wang, H., Levin-Rector, A., Dwyer, L., Costa, M., Lopez, A.D.,

Murray, C.J.L. (2010). Neonatal, Postneonatal, childhood, and under-5 mortality for 187 countries, 1970–2010: a systematic analysis of progress towards Millennium Development Goal 4. *Lancet*, Vol. 375, pp. 1988–2008.

Sachiko, B., Hiroyuki, N., Masahiro, N., Masako, W. (2011). Risk factors of early spontaneous abortions among Japanese: a matched case-control study. *Hum Reprod,*Vol.26,No.2,pp.466-72.

Sundquist, J., Sundquist, K., Johansson, S.E., Xinjun, L., Winkleby, M. (2011). Mothers, places and small for gestational age births: a cohort study. *Arch Dis Child,*Vol.96,pp.380-85.

Mumtaz, G., Nassar, A. H., Mahfoud, H., et al. (2010). Consanguinity: A risk factor for preterm births at less than 33 weeks gestation. *Am J Epidemiol,* Vol.172, pp.1424-1430.

Recape, J., De Spiegelaere, M., Alexander, S., Dramaix, M., Buekens, P., Haelterman, E. (2010). High perinatal mortality rate among immigrants in Brussles. *Eur J Public Health,* Vol. 20, No. 5, pp 536-42.

Ruan, S., Abdel-Latif, M E., Bajuk, B., Lui, K., Oel, J. L. (2011). The association between ethnicity and outcomes of infants in neonatal intensive care units. Arch Dis Child-Fetal Neonat Ed. Published on line July 2011 (213702).

Rowly, D.L., Ilyasu, S., MacDorman, M.F. Atrash, H.K. (1994). Neonatal and Post Neonatal Mortality.in Birth outcomes. From data to action. CDC's Public Health Surveillance for women, infants and children. pp 251-262. (http://www.cdc.gov/reproductivehealth/ProductsPub/dataToAction/DatatoAction.htm) Accessed September 17th 2011.

Salameh, K., Rahman, S., Al Rifai, H., Masoud, A., Lutfi, S., Adouh, G.......Bener,A. (2009). An Analytic study of trends in Perinatal and Neonatal Mortality Rates in the State of Qatar over a 30 years period (1977-2007): A comparative study with regional and developed countries. Journal of Perinatology, Vol. 29, pp. 765–770.

Salameh, K.; Rahman, S (2012). Improvements in Birth Weight-specific Neonatal Mortality Rates in the State of Qatar between 2003 and 2010 and a comparative analysis with the Vermont Oxford Network Database Report of 2007: A PEARL Study Review. JCN,Vol. 1(1),25-27.

Echer, A.I., Petterson, B., Blair, E., Ellenberg, J.H., Grether, J.K., Haan, E., Reddihough, D.S., Yeargin-Allsopp,M., Nelson, K.B. (2002). The risk of Mortality or Cerebral Palsy in Twins: A collaborative population based study. *Pediatr Res,* Vol.52, pp. 671-681.

UNICEF: State of the World's Children. (2011),pp. 89-91 (www.unicef.org) Accessed September 4th 2011.

Villadsen, S.F., Mortensen L.H., Andersen A.M.N. (2009). Ethnic disparity in stillbirth and infant mortality in Denmark 1981-2003. J Epidemiol Community Health, Vol. 63, pp. 106-12.

World Health Organization.2007.The Millennium Development Goals Report 2007. Available from: (http://www.who.org) Accessed September 10, 2011.

WHO. (2010) Word Health Statistics. (http://www.who.int/whosis/whostat/2010/en/index.html). Accessed September 4th 2011.

WHO. (2011a) Word Health Statistics. (http://www.who.int/whosis/whostat/EN_WHS2011_Full.pdf). Accessed September 4th 2011

WHO. (2011b) Indicator compendium. (http://www.who.int/whosis/indicators/en/). Accessed September 4th 2011.

Wilcox, A, J. 2001. On the importance—and the unimportance—of birth weight. *Int J Epidemiol,* Vol. 30, pp. 1233–41.

Zupan, J., Aahman, E. (2005). Perinatal Mortality for the year 2000: estimates developed by WHO, Geneva

World Health Organization. (http://www.who.int/whosis). Accessed September 5th, 2011.

Zhong-Cheng, L., Wilkins, R., Kramer, M.S., for the Fetal and Infant Health Study Group of the Canadian Perinatal Surveillance System. (2006). Effect of neighborhood income and maternal education on birth outcomes: a population study. *CMAJ,* Vol. 174, No.10,pp.Online1415-1421.

5

Perinatal Mortality in Multiple Pregnancy

Patricia Steenhaut and Corinne Hubinont
St Luc University Hospital
Belgium

1. Introduction

Twins and higher-order multiple pregnancies account for approximately 3% of all gestations in the United States (Ananth et al, 2004) and seem to be stabilized since 2006 after a dramatically increase since the beginning of the 1970s (Vayssière et al, 2011). There are two main causes for the change in the rate of multiple pregnancies: advanced maternal age and use of assisted reproductive techniques (ART) (Chauhan et al, 2010).

In occidental society, there is increasing tendency for women to delay pregnancy after 35 years. Use of fertility treatment is also more frequent in this advanced age group. The need to maximise treatment success has led to a culture of acceptance of multiple pregnancies, including high order multiples. In ART, the overall twin rate is around 26%. In the United States, the twin rate is 32%; in Latin America, it is 25%; in Europe, it is 23%; in Asia and the Middle East, it is 22%, and in Australia/New Zealand, it is 21% (Chauhan et al, 2010). Women should therefore be informed reasonably early in their childbearing years of the risks associated with late pregnancy. The perinatal mortality for multiple pregnancy exceeds that of singleton pregnancy and the optimal management should minimise losses.

2. Perinatal risks of multiple pregnancies

Health risks associated with multiple pregnancies involve both fetal and neonatal mortality. The main cause is prematurity and extreme prematurity (birth before 28 weeks gestation). The prognosis for these very preterm infants is poor, with a very low chance of intact survival if born before 26 weeks. The risk of cerebral palsy in twins has been estimated at four times that of singletons, and even moderate prematurity is associated with long term educational and behavioural problems and infant death (Black et al, 2010). Multiple pregnancies pose a number of unique challenges, such as discordant growth abnormalities, intrauterine demise, preterm premature rupture of the membranes, or premature delivery of one or both twins. At a more complex level, multiple pregnancies sharing a single placental circulation are associated with additional problems in their diagnosis and management, including twin-twin transfusion syndrome. All adverse outcomes of pregnancy, including mortality, are more likely in multiples compared with singleton pregnancies, and associated risks increase in higher order multiples.

3. Risk factors for perinatal mortality

Systematic ultrasound assessment is essential for diagnosis risk factors for fetal mortality (Hubinont et al, 2010).

3.1 Diagnosis of chorionicity and amnionicity

Chorionicity denotes the type of placentation. Monochorionic twins are always monozygotic, while dichorionic twins can be either monozygotic or dizygotic.

Diagnosis of amnionicity and chorionicity in multiple gestations is essential as monochorionic pregnancies have a greater risk for fetal morbidity and mortality than dichorionic pregnancies. The earliest and most accurate predictor for multiple gestations is the assessment of amnionicity and chorionicity. Accuracy in this diagnosis is essential, and will form the cornerstone of pregnancy counselling, decision-making, and management. Management and treatment options are now available in pregnancies with monochorionic placentation and can result in improved fetal outcome.

Every report of an ultrasound examination of a multiple pregnancy during the first trimester should include information about chorionicity and amnionicity. It is recommended that chorionicity be diagnosed as early as possible in multiple pregnancies, because the earlier the diagnosis, the more reliable it is.

During the first trimester, the most relevant signs are the number of gestational sacs between 7 and 10 weeks and the presence of a lambda sign between 11 and 14 weeks. The 'Lambda' or 'Twin peak' sign was first described by Bessis (1981) and referred to the triangular projection of tissue extending up to the base of the inter-twin membrane in dichorionic placentation. This sign is most useful in assessing pregnancies after 10 weeks. Visualization of a thin wispy membrane that comes to a T-shape 90° junction at the base indicates the presence of a diamniotic-monochorionic gestation.

In dichorionic twin pregnancy, the intertwin membrane includes two chorion layers interposed between amnion. Thus a thick intertwin membrane is more likely to be seen in dichorionic than a monochorionic-diamniotic twin pregnancy.

Sensitivity for determining chorionicity based on membrane thickness declines with increasing gestation. There is no clear cut-off for membrane thickness, although several studies reported a 2 mm cut-off, while others suggest a lower cut-off of 1.5 mm. The absence of any dividing membrane on repeated investigations, the absence of a T-sign, and the presence of a single yolk sac are associated with a monochorionic-monoamniotic gestation.

Two separate placentas or gender discordance ensures dichorionicity of the twin pregnancies, but the converse is not always true. Dichorionic twin pregnancies can be of the same gender and a single placenta could be the result of two contiguous fused placenta of a dichorionic twin pregnancy.

Membrane analysis in the second trimester is similar to that performed in the first trimester for thickness and the presence of either the twin-peak or T-shaped sign. Many authors have reported that chorionicity assessment is less accurate in second and third trimester. After 20 weeks of gestation the 'twin-peak sign' disappeared in about 7% of dichorionic pregnancies due to regression of the chorion frondosum (Sepulveda et al, 1997).

The number of layers in the dividing membrane can also be used to assess chorionicity; however it is not particularly helpful. The inter-fetal membrane needs to be magnified under high resolution and ideally perpendicular to the ultrasound probe to identify the number of layers.

If chorionicity is appropriately diagnosed during the first trimester of pregnancy and the 'explicit photograph of the ultrasound image allowing diagnosis of chorionicity' can be available, this diagnosis should not to be reconsidered later.

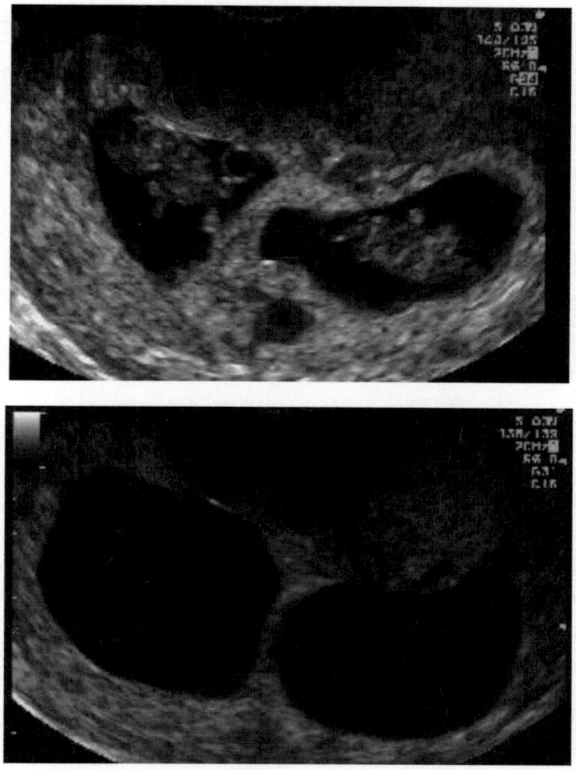

Fig. 1. Chorionicity determination in the first trimester. Ultrasound images of dichorionic pregnancies. The 'full' lambda sign reflects the apposition of the two placental disks.

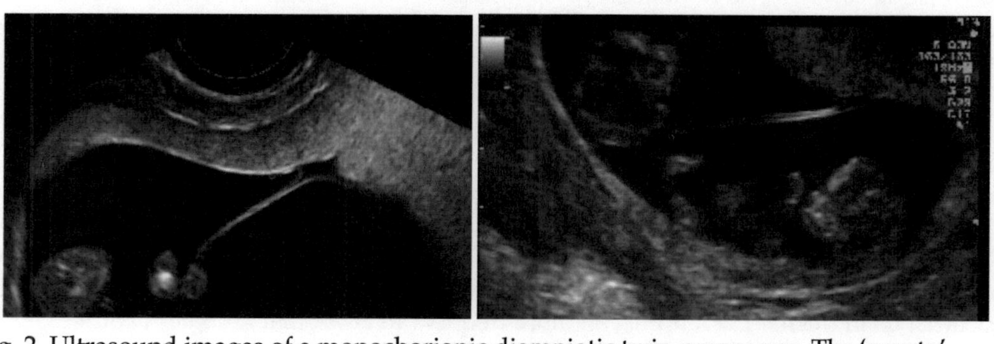

Fig. 2. Ultrasound images of a monochorionic diamniotic twin pregnancy. The 'empty' lambda sign or the T sign: only two thin layers of amniotic membranes separate the twins.

3.2 Congenital malformations

Twin pregnancies have an increased risk of congenital malformations, especially monochorionic twins (Sperling et al, 2007). Congenital anomalies may be the result of the teratogenic insult responsible for the twinning. For any given defect in a twin pregnancy, the pregnancy may be concordant or discordant, although the majority of structural defect are discordant, regardless of zygosity. Discordance in non-identical (dizygotic) twins is usually due to differences in genetic predisposition, whereas in identical (monozygotic twins) twins, it may be a consequence of the underlying stimulus to zygote splitting, variation in gene expression, or abnormal placentation (Hendrix et al, 1998).

Structural anomalies have been reported to occur more often in monozygotic twins with relative risks of congenital anomalies in twins compared with singletons of 1.17 for dizygotic twins (Myrianthopoulos et al, 1978) and 1.25 for monozygotic twins (Mastroiacovo et al, 1999). Major congenital defects are found in about 6% of twin pregnancies and usually, only one twin is affected (Lewi et al, 2007). Cardiac anomalies are significantly prevalent amongst monochorionic twins (Manning et al, 2006 and Bahtiyar et al, 2007). The incidence of congenital malformations was 3.2% among monozygotic and 2.2% among dizygotic twins. Cardiac abnormalities accounted for 68% of all abnormalities (Sperling et al, 2007).

3.3 Aneuploidy screening

3.3.1 Maternal serum markers

Serum screening is of limited value in twin pregnancies because the mean sensitivity is associated with a high false-positive rate and the screening test does not provide the separate risk for each fetus. Screening in twin pregnancies requires adjustment of the multiple of the median (MoM) to account for the presence of two fetuses. Different factors are required for the observed corrected MoM for free β human chorionic gonadotropin and pregnancy-associated plasma protein-A (Spencer et al, 2008). The routine use of serum markers during first trimester is not recommended but their use is currently being assessed (Vayssière et al, 2011)

3.3.2 Nuchal translucency (NT)

Enlarged nuchal translucency appears in fetuses affected by pathological conditions such as some chromosomal abnormalities, congenital heart defects, major extracardiac malformations and genetic syndromes. In singleton pregnancies, enlarged nuchal translucency (greater than the 95th centile) is encountered in about 5% of cases and in dichorionic pregnancies the frequency is about the same. In fetuses of monochorionic diamniotic pregnancies the frequency of an enlarged nuchal translucency is significantly higher, about 15%, without epidemiological demonstration of a higher frequency of chromosomal abnormalities (Sebire et al, 2000). In a monochorionic pregnancy, in which fetuses share the same placenta, enlarged nuchal translucency may affect one or both fetuses. First-trimester imbalance in the placental circulation between the two fetal compartments may be one of the causes of the nuchal translucency enlargement. Discordance in nuchal translucency is more frequent in cases that are later complicated by twin-to-twin transfusion syndrome or have an unfavourable outcome. The risk of developing severe TTTS requiring fetoscopic laser surgery can be predicted from the intertwin discordance in fetal nuchal translucency at 11 to 13 + 6 weeks. The risk is more than 30% in those pregnancies with discordance in nuchal translucency of 20% or more, compared to less than 10% in those with a smaller discordance (Kagan et al, 2007). Nuchal translucency enlargement may also be attributable to the presence of fetal structural defects especially cardiac defects (Bahtiyar et al, 2007). When enlarged nuchal translucency is found in both fetuses, the presence of an abnormal karyotype may be the underlying pathological condition. Discordance in nuchal translucency and discrepant karyotype (heterokaryotypia) may result from a mitotic error arising after splitting and resulting in the chromosomal abnormality only in one of the fetuses. Although the frequency of heterokaryotypia is very low, this possibility should be kept in mind when a discordant nuchal translucency thickness is found (Cheng et al, 2006).

4. Complications and contribution of multiple pregnancies to the burden perinatal mortality

4.1 Preterm delivery

Twins are more likely to be delivered preterm (< 37 weeks of gestation) than singletons. In 2006, in the United States, approximately 60% of the twins were preterm and weighed less than 2500g. Approximately 1 out of 10 twin was born at below 32 weeks of gestation or weighed less than 1500g (Chauhan et al, 2010). The perinatal mortality in twins is related to comorbidity factors such as premature rupture of membranes, socioeconomical and ethnical factors, gestational age, fetal gender and availability of antenatal management with corticosteroids. In some complicated and high-risk twins pregnancies, elective preterm birth is indicated to avoid specific complications described later.

4.2 Complications of monochorionicity

Monochorionic twins account for 20% of spontaneous twin pregnancies and almost 5% occur as a result of assisted reproductive techniques (Cordero et al, 2005). The incidence of monochorionic twin pregnancies is increasing, as there are more pregnancies in older women associated with twins (Aston et al, 2008).

These fetuses are at higher risks of adverse outcome, compared with dichorionic twins and singleton pregnancies. The main reason for this is an unbalanced flow in the placental vascular anastomoses connecting both fetal circulations. Vascular complications in monochorionic twins are well known and may cause different disorders. The most important is twin-twin transfusion syndrome (TTTS), complicated around 10-15% of twins with monochorionic placentation. Other complications include growth retardation, twin anemia polycythemia sequence, twin reversed arterial perfusion, congenital heart disease due to vascular instability, fetal demise, and long-term neonatal and pediatric morbidity secondary to vascular insults in fetal brain, heart and kidneys (Lewi et al, 2010). Vascular disruptive sequences cumulating in TTTS can include infarction of the intestine or skin resulting in widespread skin aplasia or intestinal atresia, or infarction of the brain, kidneys, liver and lungs (Sperling et al, 2007).

A recent systematic review demonstrated that the incidence of congenital heart malformations is about 5%, some 9-fold higher than expected for a singleton pregnancy.

Given this last observation (Bahtiyar et al, 2007), detailed echocardiography would seem to be an appropriate routine investigation in all monochorionic pregnancies.

4.2.1 Twin-to-twin transfusion syndrome (TTTS)

TTTS, also called twin oligoamnios polyhydramnios sequence (TOPS), complicates around 15% of monochorionic pregnancies irrespective of the mode of conception. It is a hemodynamic, and probably hormonal, discordance secondary to imbalanced blood flow through the vascular anastomoses (Hubinont et Fisk, 1990) (Chalouhi et al, 2011). The natural history of untreated TTTS leads to intra- or perinatal death in 90% of cases (Robyr et al, 2006). Impaired neurological development is reported in up to 50% of survivors as a consequence of prematurity or the intrauterine fetal demise of one twin (Haverkamp et al, 2001).

TTTS can be diagnosed at any time in gestation. Membrane folding or intertwin disparity in fetal growth, nuchal translucency thickness or amniotic fluid volumes are early signs of the possible development of TTTS and indicate the need for increased ultrasound surveillance of monochorionic pregnancies. This syndrome can also be suspected by acute maternal symptoms related to polyhydramnios (uterine distension, uterine contractions, dyspnea) (Chalouhi et al, 2011).

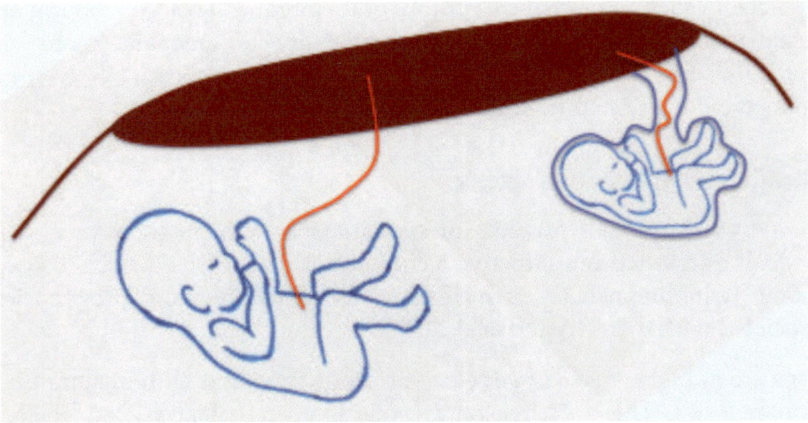

Fig. 3. 'Stuck twin' in a TTTS in a monochorionic diamniotic twin pregnancy.

The diagnosis relies upon strict ultrasound criteria as defined in the Eurofetus trial (Senat et al, 2004) and consist of a polyuric polyhydramnios in the recipient twin with a deepest vertical pool of at least 8.0 cm at or before 20 weeks of gestation or 10.0 cm after 20 weeks of gestation together with a distended fetal bladder, with oliguric oligohydramnios in the donor twin, showing a deepest vertical pool of at most 2.0 cm. Ultrasound staging of TTTS was introduced in 1999 by Quintero and provided a reproductible classification.

TTTS may also occurs in monoamniotic twins. In these patients, the absence of a dividing membrane does not allow development of oligohydramnios in the donor. Rather, the single amniotic cavity has polyhydramnios. The diagnosis is made by noting polyhydramnios and differences in bladder filling or Doppler studies.

Stage	Poly/oligo Hydramnios	Absent bladder in the donor	Abnormal Dopplers flow	Hydrops	Demise
I	+	-	-	-	-
II	+	+	-	-	-
III	+	+	+	-	-
IV	+	+	+	+	-
V	+	+	+	+	+

Table 1. Quintero staging of TTTS based on sonographic and Doppler findings (Quintero et al, 1999)

The prognosis is not accurately related to the Quintero's staging because the natural history of TTTS does not follow an orderly progression through the stages over time. A number of 'early stage' cases do not progress and remain at stage 1 or even regress. As Quintero's staging does not take into account the fundamental cardiovascular perturbations, recent articles have focused on the value of the recipient's cardiac function (Barrea et al, 2006). This has led to the development of independent scoring systems based upon echocardiographic and peripheral Doppler findings. Rychik et al (2007) proposed the Children's Hospital of Philadelphia scoring system, designed to represent the cardiovascular status of the twins and which correlated with the Quintero staging system. Shah et al (2008) designed a very similar scoring system with the cardiovascular profile score. Stirnemann et al (2010) developed cardiac profiling allowing discrimination of cases with significant myocardial dysfunction as well as assessment of the severity of the recipient's cardiomyopathy.

4.2.2 Twin anemia polycythemia sequence (TAPS)

Twin anemia-polycythemia sequence (TAPS) is an atypical form of twin-twin transfusion syndrome. There is a large intertwin hemoglobin difference with one twin developing chronic anemia with reticulocytosis and the other developing polycythemia, without oligohydramnios-polyhydramnios sequence (Lopriore et al, 2007). The prenatal diagnostic criteria for TAPS require that the middle cerebral artery-peak systolic velocity (MCA-PSV) measure greater than 1.5 multiples of median (MoM) in the donor twin and less than 0.08 MoM in the recipient twin (Robyr et al, 2006). A chronic rather than an acute intertwin transfusion is diagnosed by an elevated reticulocyte count in the anemic twin. The presumed etiology of TAPS involves the presence of small unidirectional artery-to-vein anastomoses, suggesting that TAPS results from a chronic net transfusion across these tiny anastomoses. TAPS can occur spontaneously in about 5% of previously uncomplicated monochorionic pregnancies. It is, however better known in its iatrogenic form as a complication of incomplete laser treatment for TTTS. TAPS begins usually after 30 weeks, especially in pairs with late-onset discordant growth (Lewi et al, 2007). Because of its late presentation, the mortality of TAPS is likely to be lower than that of TTTS (Lewi et al, 2010). Symptomatic treatment consists of intrauterine transfusion of the anemic twin combined eventually with hemodilution of the polycythemic co-twin. Laser therapy was used as causative treatment to interrupt the shared circulation. Selective feticide by cord occlusion can be offered in cases with severe associated anomalies (Gucciardo et al, 2010)

4.2.3 Selective intrauterine growth restriction

Selective intrauterine growth restriction (sIUGR) is a common condition associated with monochorionic pregnancy. It is increasingly considered to be an important complication of monochorionic twins, with potentially significant risks of intrauterine fetal demise or neurological adverse outcome for both twins (Lewi et al, 2008).

The term 'selective intrauterine growth restriction' in monochorionic pregnancies is applicable to cases where the estimated fetal weight (EFW) of the small fetus falls below the 10th percentile. Significant fetal weight discordance is an important element of the clinical picture, which will often accompany this condition, but is not necessary for diagnosis. Fetal weight discordance is defined as a difference between the EFW of two fetuses > 25% and is calculated as the difference between the EFW of the larger twin and the smaller twin divided by the EFW of the larger twin. The prevalence of sIUGR based on an EFW below the 10th percentile ranges from 10 to 15%. However, in contrast to TTTS, it has a much lower mortality, about 10 versus 55% (Lewi et al, 2007).

The most feared complication of sIUGR is the intrauterine demise of the growth-restricted twin. However substantial risks for the normally grown twin are well known even if both fetuses are born alive. These risks stem from two main factors. First, since these pregnancies must by definition be delivered before the death of the IUGR fetus, the normal twin is exposed to severe prematurity with its known consequences in terms of neurodevelopmental sequelae. Second, even if prematurity is avoided, there may be an increased prevalence of neurological complications in the normally grown twin due to a high risk of acute feto-fetal transfusion accidents in utero (Ishii et al, 2009). The specific risks for these two complications may vary in different types of sIUGR, as discussed later.

The principle cause for the development of sIUGR in monochorionic twins is inadequate placental sharing. Aside from placental territory discordance, a second factor largely influencing fetal weight discordance and the natural history of sIUGR in monochorionic twins is the presence of vascular anastomoses in the monochorionic placenta (Lewi et al, 2007). The presence of placental anastomoses has a protective effect on the IUGR fetus, which receives blood from its co-twin that may partially compensate the placental insufficiency.

As a consequence of the combination of the effects of placental insufficiency with those of the inter-twin vascular connections, monochorionic pregnancies with similar degrees of fetal weight discordance may be associated with remarkable differences in clinical course and outcome. The identification of groups with similar clinical behavior may facilitate clinical management. To date, the clinical technique that best achieves this goal is umbilical artery (UA) Doppler of the IUGR twin.

A classification system of sIUGR is established into three types according to the umbilical artery Doppler patterns in the fetus with IUGR. Accordingly, pregnancies are defined as type I (normal umbilical artery Doppler), type II (persistent absent or reversed end-diastolic flow, AREDF) or type III (intermittently absent or reversed end-diastolic flow, iARED). This classification may help to understand and predict the distinct clinical evolutions and to plan clinical management of the different clinical forms of sIUGR (Valsky et al, 2010).

4.2.3.1 Type I sIUGR

The type I Doppler pattern is distinguished by positive diastolic flow in the umbilical artery of the small twin.

Types I cases are generally associated with good outcomes with intrauterine mortality rates of 2-4% (Gratacos et al, 2007). As clinical evolution of sIUGR type I cases has been shown to be benign in most cases, a policy of expectant management and close follow-up to rule out progression to type II Doppler patterns seems reasonable. In the absence of such progression, bi-weekly sonographic and Doppler surveillance could be proposed. In most cases, the IUGR fetus will remain with a normal Doppler until advanced stages of pregnancy allowing elective delivery, which can be performed at around 34-35 weeks (Valsky et al, 2010).

4.2.3.2 Type II sIUGR

Type II pattern is characterized by persistently absent or reversed end-diastolic flow (AREDF) in the umbilical artery.

Unlike type I, the great majority sIUGR type II will show in utero deterioration, but with important differences with respect to singletons or dichorionic twins. Type II sIUGR shows a remarkably longer latency time between the onset of AREDF and delivery, on average 10 weeks, compared with the 3-4 weeks reported in singletons with IUGR and similar findings in the UA Doppler (Vanderheyden et al, 2005). Severe fetal deterioration, as defined by abnormal venous Doppler or biophysical profile, will occur in the majority of type II cases (Gratacos et al, 2007). Elective delivery is indicated in most of these pregnancies earlier than 30 weeks of gestation (Gratacos et al, 2007) with only a small minority surviving in utero beyond 32 weeks. Thus, placental insufficiency in type II is far more severe than in type I and cannot be fully compensated by inter-twin transfusion. In 2007, Gratacos et al reported the outcome of 30 type II pregnancies, showing an extremely high deterioration rate (90%), as defined by abnormal venous Dopplers or biophysical profile. Mean gestational age at delivery was 30 weeks and the rate of neonatal brain damage of the small twin was 15%. In 2009, Ishii et al reported the outcome of 27 type II pregnancies. Intrauterine death occurred in 30% among IUGR twins and 22% among larger twins. The rate of neonatal brain damage of the small twin at 6 months was 15%. Mean gestational age at delivery was 28 weeks. The latency time between diagnosis of AREDF and fetal deterioration may be long and UA Doppler cannot be used as a predictor of imminent fetal death. The abnormal ductus venosus defined by absent or reversed atrial flow can be used as a criterion suggesting imminent fetal demise and indicating selective feticide or delivery to prevent the occurrence of in utero death (Gratacos et al, 2007). A weekly follow-up scheme may be reasonable if venous Doppler is normal, and a more frequent follow-up when venous Doppler pulsatility index becomes abnormal. Biophysical profile can be included in the follow-up protocol after viability is reached. Management options depend on gestational age and the severity of growth restriction. Fetal therapy should be contemplated to protect the larger twin from the death of its co-twin if deterioration occurs before viability is reached. Cord occlusion is the most straightforward and less risky procedure (Valsky et al, 2010).

4.2.3.3 Type III sIUGR

Type III is defined by the presence of intermittent absent or reversed end-diastolic flow (iAREDF) in the umbilical artery Doppler of the IUGR twin. The characteristic feature of this Doppler pattern is the alternation of phases of positive with phases of absent or reversed diastolic flow, normally but not always in a cyclical fashion. The observation of this sign indicates the presence of a large placental arterio-arterial (AA) anastomosis (Gratacos et al, 2004).

Contrary to type I cases these pregnancies are associated with a significant increase in the risk of unexpected intrauterine fetal demise of the IUGR fetus and of brain injury in the normally grown twin. These adverse outcomes are explained by the high risk of acute feto-fetal hemorrhagic accidents through the large AA vessel, which may lead to death of the smaller twin or acute hypovolemia in the larger one. Such acute feto-fetal transfusion may occur in the presence of short episode of bradycardia or hypotension in the smaller twin, and are facilitated by the large diameter of the AA anastomosis, which facilitates direct and rapid transfusion over a period of seconds (Valsky et al, 2010).

The majority of type III IUGR fetuses progresses until 32 weeks or later without abnormal venous Doppler or biophysical profile changes suggestive of fetal deterioration. In spite of this apparently benign evolution, 15% of IUGR fetuses die unexpectedly hours or days after a normal examination. In addition, even if both twins are alive, the larger twin had a significantly increased incidence (19%) of abnormal neonatal brain scans (Valsky et al, 2010).

Management of type III sIUGR represents a challenge (Valsky et al, 2010). Left to its natural evolution the prognosis would be better than in type II cases, but clinical decisions are more difficult due to the unpredictability of adverse outcomes. If expectant management is chosen, follow-up schemes should be similar to these discussed for type II cases; weekly follow-up if venous Doppler is normal, and closer follow-up with consideration of active management if venous Doppler becomes abnormal. Unfortunately, in type III the IUGR fetus will rarely show signs of fetal deterioration in venous Doppler, and therefore one reasonable option may be to deliver electively around 32 weeks of gestation. The reasons are similar to those used for decisions in monoamniotic pregnancies: to reduce the opportunity for unexpected adverse outcomes to occur. Type III pregnancies with milder forms of intermittent absent end-diastolic flow and moderate EFW discordance could probably be prolonged until 34 weeks. In case fetal therapy is considered, cord occlusion is a straightforward treatment. It seems reasonable that this therapy should normally be reserved for cases with extreme forms of iAREDF and/or extreme EFW discordance, or if fetal deterioration of the IUGR fetus is observed.

4.2.4 Twin reversed arterial perfusion (TRAP) sequence

TRAP is an abnormality unique to monochorionic twins with an estimated prevalence of approximately 1 in 35.000 pregnancies. In TRAP, the acardiac twin is a true parasite receiving blood from the pump twin through an arterioarterial anastomosis. The condition is associated with a high risk of perinatal death of the pump twin caused by a combination of high-output cardiac failure and polyhydramnios-related preterm birth (Moore et al, 1990).

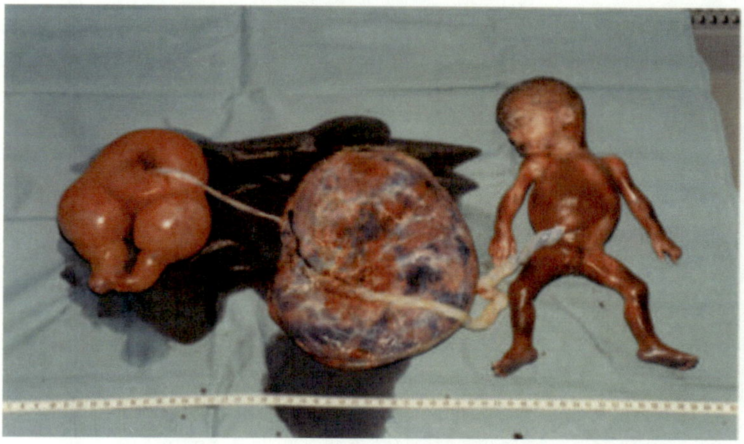

Fig. 4. Monochorionic twins pregnancy complicated by TRAP sequence.

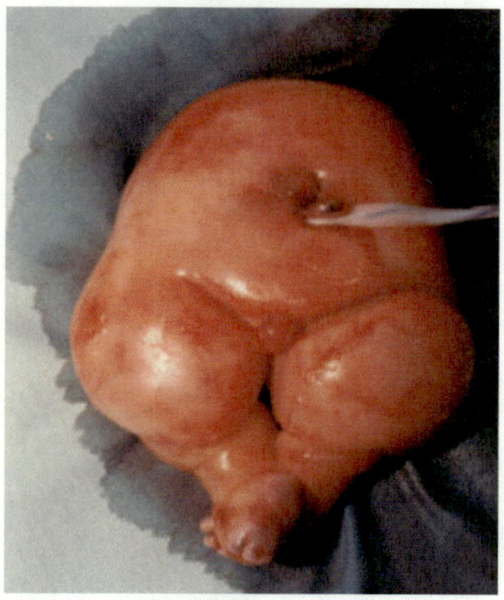

Fig. 5. Acardiac twin in a TRAP sequence.

The outcome may be improved by intrauterine intervention to arrest the circulation of the acardiac twin, as described below. In 33% of pregnancies, spontaneous death of the pump twin occurs between diagnosis and planned intervention. In 21%, there is a spontaneous arrest of flow (Lewi et al, 2010).

4.2.5 Monoamniotic twins

Monochorionic monoamniotic twins represents approximately 1% of all monozygous twins (Dickinson et al, 2005). Monoamniotic twins are the result of ovum division beyond 8 days postconception and are characterized by a single amnion and a single yolk sac. There may be two or one (conjoined twins) embryos present.

4.2.5.1 Conjoined twins

Conjoined twinning arises when the twinning event occurs at about 13-14 days after fertilization. Conjoined twinning occurs by the incomplete splitting of the embryonic axis.

Conjoined twins are typically classified by the point at which their bodies are joined. Management could be based on early assessment of fetal sharing by ultrasound and fetoscopy (Hubinont et al, 1997).

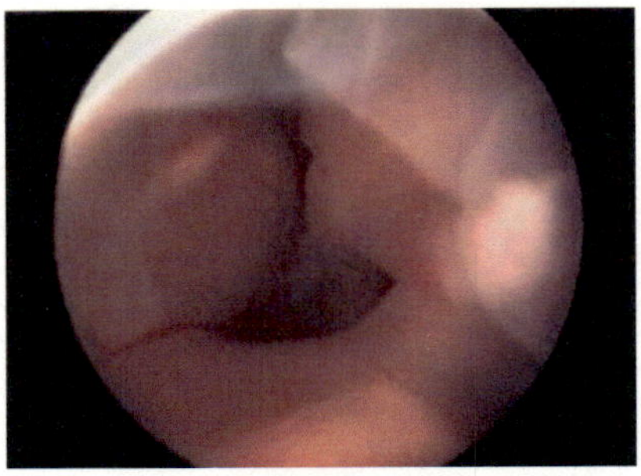

Fig. 6. Fetoscopic image of conjoined twins (Hubinont et al, 1997).

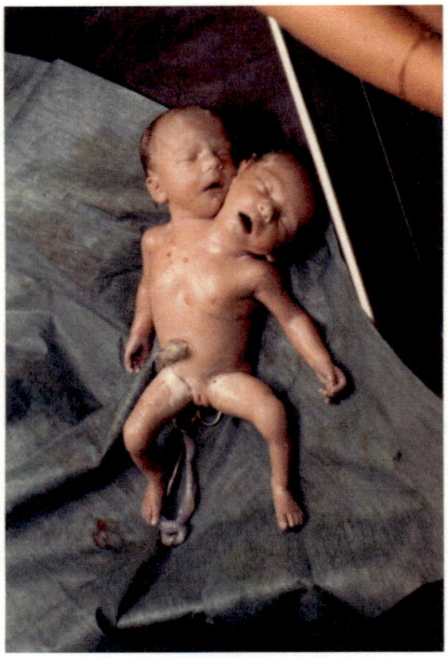

Fig. 7. Dicephalus: unusual case of conjoined twins (Hubinont et al, 1984).

4.2.5.2 Cord entanglement in monoamniotic twins

In monoamniotic twins, the high perinatal mortality rates have been attributed mainly to umbilical cord entanglement, intertwin transfusion syndromes, discordant fetal abnormality or growth restriction. Fetal demise because of umbilical cord entanglement and secondary cord occlusion is a unique characteristic of monoamniotic twin pregnancies. Umbilical cord entanglement is present in the great majority of monoamniotic twin pregnancies and may result in dual or single fetal demise. Umbilical cord entanglement may be detected with prenatal ultrasound and color Doppler. The initiation of cord entanglement can occur as early as first trimester, when the amniotic fluid volume in relation to the fetal mass is greater (Arabin et al 1999). In the literature, many strategies have been proposed including admission to hospital - after viability has been established - with cardiotocography several times a day and the use of pharmacological agents to reduce amniotic fluid volume in the hope of preventing fetal loss from cord accidents. Intensive cardiotocographic monitoring may prevent some fetal deaths, but it is not surprising that it does not prevent all intrauterine death, as cord accidents can occur acutely without prior warning. Medical amnioreduction with sulindac, a non-selective prostaglandine synthase inhibitor used to treat preterm labor and polyhydramnios, was described to prevent the accumulation of a relative abundance of amniotic fluid that would otherwise allow unrestricted fetal movements and changes in fetal position, which contribute to the high intrauterine death rate from cord entanglement, compression and/or tightening of cord knots (Pasquini et al, 2006).

The cumulative rates of cord entanglement and perinatal mortality in the recent literature are 74% and 21% respectively (Table 1).

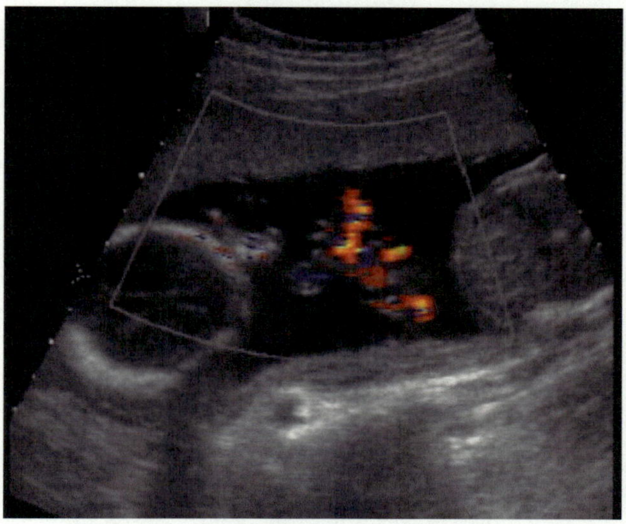

Fig. 8. Ultrasound image and color Doppler showing umbilical cord entanglement in a monoamniotic twin pregnancy.

Reference	Number of cases	Cord entanglement (n(%))	Intrauterine death (n)	Survivors (n)	Perinatal survival rate (%)
Sau et al. 2003	7	4 (57)	5	9	64
Ezra el al. 2005	30	26 (87)	24	35	58
Cordero et al. 2006	36	15 (42)	1	66	92
Pasquini et al. 2006	20	19 (95)	0	40	100
Hack et al. 2009	98	Not reported	34	150	77
Dias et al. 2010	18	18 (100)	2	32	89
Total	209	82/111 (74)		332/418	79

Table 2. Review of the published literature since 2000 indicating prevalence of cord entanglement and perinatal outcome (Dias et al, 2010).

4.3 Management of a twin pregnancy after in utero death

Single fetal death in a twin pregnancy is known to be a serious complication of pregnancy. It is a relatively rare complication of multiple pregnancies (6,2% of all twin pregnancies, Hillman et al, 2010) but may carry with its increased risk of perinatal morbidity and mortality.

Single intrauterine death can lead to adverse outcomes on the surviving co-twins, especially in monochorionic pregnancies. Co-twin death, neurological damage and preterm delivery have been reported as potential complications of these pregnancies. Surviving twins of dichorionic pregnancies develop fewer complications mainly due to prematurity, whereas those of monochorionic twins sets are also at greater risk of perinatal death or significant sequelae. In monochorionic pregnancies, placental anastomoses account for the poor outcome of the surviving twin (Ong et al, 2006). Two theories have been advanced to explain severe sequelae and co-twin death in these pregnancies. The first is that there is passage of thrombotic materiel from the dead to healthy twin following derangement in coagulation due to the death of one twin (Benirschke et al, 1993). The second theory states that the placental anastomoses allow transfer of blood from the surviving twin to the dead co-twin giving rise to periods of hypoperfusion, hypotension and acute fetal anemia, resulting in neurological damage (Bajoria et al, 1997). If the hypovolemic episode is severe, the surviving twin may develop ischemic lesions in vital organs such as the brain and the kidneys or, in some cases, die from hypovolemic shock or parenchymal damage.

It has been suggested that the possible mechanism responsible for organ damages or death of monochorionic co-twins occur probably before or at the time of single death and no therapeutic strategies after the diagnosis of death have been clearly demonstrated to reduce the risks of adverse outcome (Fichera et al, 2009).

Current practice advocates an expectant approach by serial fetal ultrasound and cerebral magnetic resonance imaging (MRI). An intensive surveillance in the 1-4 weeks following the diagnosis of intrauterine death is recommended to exclude cerebral lesions in utero and subsequent neurological sequelae in surviving monochorionic co-twins (Hillman et al, 2010).

Given this sequence of events in the death of monochorionic twins, conservative management has been advocated as the option of choice to avoid the risks of prematurity and therefore immediate delivery is an ineffective strategy to prevent co-twin damage (Nicolini et al, 1999).

A recent study (Fichera et al, 2009) confirmed the trend to an increased risk of perinatal mortality for the co-twin in case of single intrauterine death. This study reported a risk of co-twin death in utero of 16,5% for monochorionic pregnancies. A systematic review reported a risk of 18% of neurological sequelae in these cases (Ong et al, 2006).

5. Preconceptional prevention of multiple pregnancy related perinatal mortality

One of the priorities in the management of infertile couples remains the prevention of twin and higher-order multiple pregnancies in assisted reproductive techniques (ART). Attempts at reducing the incidence of higher-order multiples, such as triplets or more, have met with some success in countries that have legislated against multiple embryo reimplantations during in vitro fertilization (IVF) cycles. However, even in these tightly controlled cycles twin pregnancies occur at a rate 10-fold that of normal cycle conception (Wimalasundera et al, 2003).

6. Antenatal prevention of multiple pregnancy related perinatal mortality

6.1 Selective termination of severely affected twin and multifetal pregnancy reduction

In the case of a discordant aneuploidy or an especially severe malformation of a twin, a selective feticide can be performed as early as the end of the first trimester. A multifetal pregnancy reduction can also be performed in patients with high-order multiple gestations in an effort to improve perinatal survival. Techniques should be chosen according to chorionicity.

6.1.1 Dichorionic twins

In dichorionic twins, selective pregnancy reduction or feticide are possible by potassium chloride intracardiac administration and do not present a direct risk to the healthy twin (Evans et al, 2004).

6.1.2 Monochorionic twins

In monochorionic pregnancies, a selective termination requires special considerations. The acute blood loss into the vascular anastomoses can cause death or severe neurologic impairment of the remaining unaffected twin. Selective feticide by umbilical cord occlusion is performed with bipolar forceps to prevent co-twin death and transfusional tissue injury. In the absence of imminent risk for the healthy twin, this procedure is recommended at or after 18 weeks. The risk of premature rupture of the membranes is approximately 20% and survival around 80% of the other twin (Vayssière et al, 2011).

Recent advances in vascular-occlusive techniques have allowed the possibility of selective termination in monochorionic pregnancies in the presence of discordant anomalies or multifetal reduction with radiofrequency ablation and cord occlusion appearing to be the most successful (Wimalasundera et al, 2010).

In early gestation intra-fetal techniques including interstitial laser and radiofrequency are used. Pregnancy loss and prematurity are the main risks of selective feticide and fetal reduction. Such complications have decreased as experience with the procedure has grown (Evans et al, 2005).

6.2 Invasive fetal therapy in monochorionic complications

TTTS is clinically characterized by an acute polyhydramnios (uterine distension, uterine contractions, dyspnea) causing maternal discomfort with an increased risk for preterm labor and premature rupture of the membranes.

6.2.1 Amnioreduction

One of the first treatments implemented for TTTS was serial therapeutic amnioreductions. The rationale for this technique is to prevent preterm labor related to polyhydramnios. It was also hypothesized that amnioreduction may improve fetal hemodynamics by decreasing pressure on the placental surface vasculature (Elliott et al, 1991). Therapeutic amnioreduction has the great advantage to be a simple technique but has the disadvantage to require multiple procedures in the majority of cases (Hubinont et al, 2000).

6.2.2 Septostomy

Septostomy involves intentional puncture or rupture of the inter-twin septum and was first reported by our team on the occasion of a case that did improve following unintentional septostomy (Hubinont et al, 1996). The proposed mechanism of septostomy in TTTS is to equilibrate amniotic fluid pressure and maybe to provide available amniotic fluid around the donor and improve fetal hemodynamics. The main specific additional risk is the iatrogenic creation of a pseudo-monoamniotic twin pregnancy that can lead to cord entanglement. However, this may be reduced by performing a small hole just as in transeptal diagnostic amniocentesis in twins. Another potential risk of septostomy is to create floating amniotic membranes that could induce amniotic band syndrome (Hubinont et al, 2000).

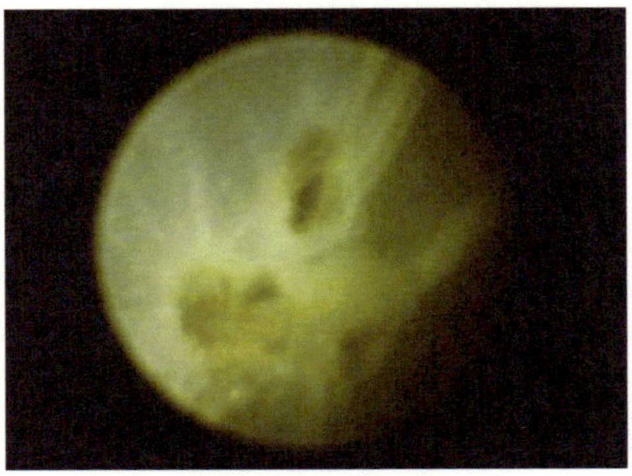

Fig. 9. Fetoscopic image of intertwin septostomy in TTTS.

6.2.3 Laser coagulation

Fetoscopic (selective) laser coagulation of the placental vascular anastomoses is currently the best available treatment for TTTS diagnosed before 26 weeks. In the Eurofetus randomized controlled trial, Senat et al (2004) compared the safety and efficacy of laser surgery and amnioreduction in TTTS diagnosed between 15 and 26 weeks; endoscopic laser treatment resulted in a higher likelihood ratio of survival of at least one twin, and a smaller risk of neurological complications in the infant at 6 months of age. The risks of brain injury are reduced after fetoscopic placental laser but incompletely prevented in cases of incomplete coagulation of vascular anastomoses. Whereas previous data had shown a benefit of laser treatment only in foetuses with Stages 3 and 4, Senat also found a better outcome for fetuses with Stages 1 and 2. After 26 weeks, TTTS could be managed by amniodrainage, elective preterm delivery and in particularly sick twin by selective cord coagulation.

At the present time, amnioreduction is no longer the treatment of choice for pregnancies complicated by TTTS. It may still have a role in the management of TTTS under certain conditions. For example, to allow a patient to be transported to a center where laser may be offered, to decompress the uterus before a cerclage (in case of cervical shortening), to manage symptomatic polyhydramnios when TTTS develops outside the gestational age when laser can be performed or when laser is technically not possible and finally, potentially, to manage stage I TTTS (Fichera et al, 2010).

It is important to recognize signs of TTTS early to improve the management of these pregnancies and diminish fetal loss and infant mortality rate among twins. Twice-monthly ultrasound monitoring, sometimes even weekly, is recommended for this type of pregnancy. TTTS is an obstetric emergency that is easy to diagnose with ultrasound. Treatment and counselling must be performed in a center that can offer fetoscopic laser coagulation of placental anastomoses. Monitoring after treatment should be conducted in association with the reference center. In the absence of complications after laser treatment, planned delivery is recommended from 34 weeks and no later than 37 weeks.

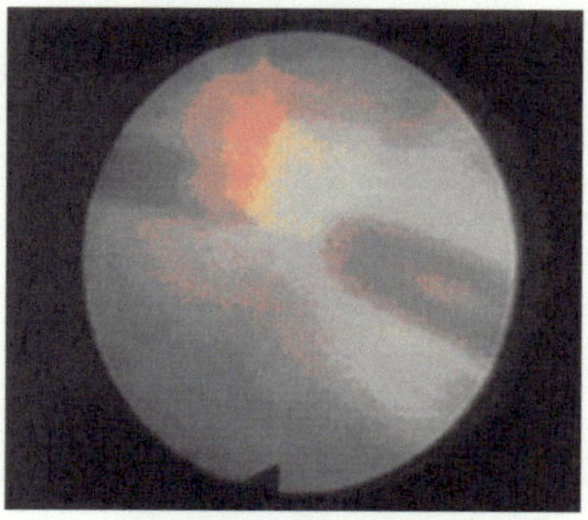

Fig. 10. Fetoscopic image of laser coagulation of the placental vascular anastomoses.

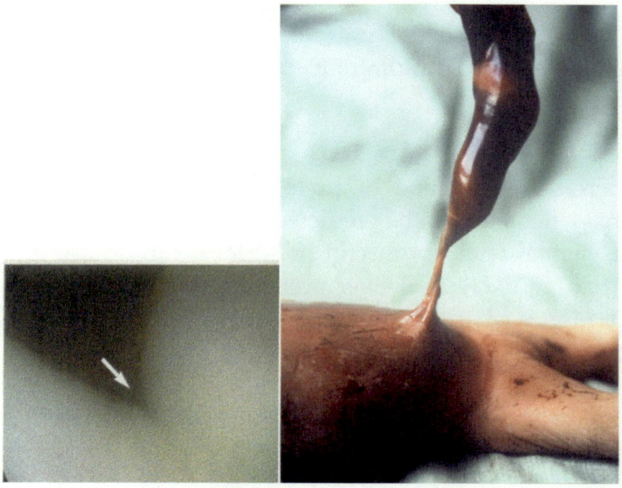

Fig. 11. Fetoscopic image of selective cord occlusion in a TTTS. Selective feticide by cord coagulation.

In twin reversed arterial perfusion (TRAP) sequence, the technique used to arrest the flow toward the acardiac twin consists of either ultrasound-guided intrafetal coagulation or fetoscopic laser coagulation of the umbilical cord and/or placental anastomoses. Intrafetal coagulation can be performed by using a radiofrequency needle (Livingston et al, 2007). Prophylactic surgery at 16-18 weeks seems to be the best option. Intrauterine interventions are performed after 16 weeks (after obliteration of the celomic cavity) to reduce the risk of miscarriage. It seems preferable not to await signs of cardiac failure in the pump twin. Prophylactic intervention precludes the difficulty of achieving arrest of flow in the larger and often hydropic acardiac mass later on in pregnancy. In the patients undergoing prophylactic surgery at 16-18 weeks, 90% of infants survived and in 90% delivery was after 32 weeks (Lewi et al, 2010).

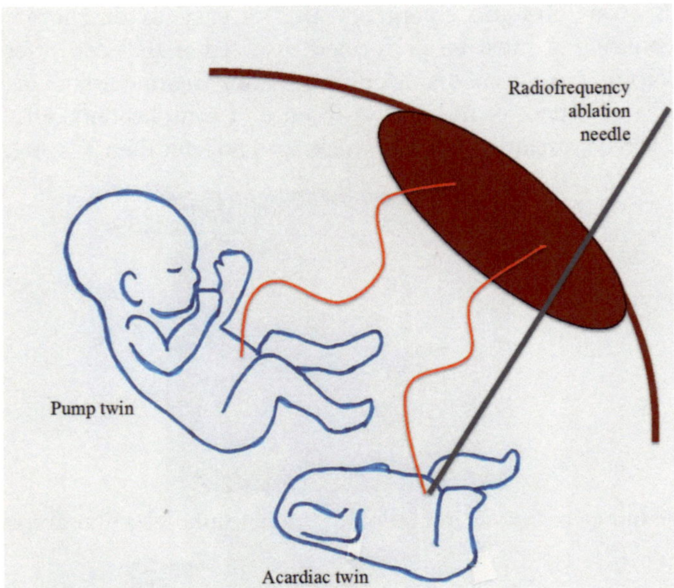

Fig. 12. Intrauterine intervention by radiofrequency ablation in a TRAP sequence.

6.3 Management of preterm birth

Considering the increased likelihood of preterm births among twin pregnancies, it is essential to determine whether it can be predicted. Transvaginal ultrasound measurement of cervical length and vaginal fetal fibronectin (fFN) level can be useful tool to differentiate those pregnancies that are likely to deliver prematurely. The rate of spontaneous preterm birth is significantly higher when either fFN is positive and/or cervical length is < 20 mm (Chauhan et al, 2010).

6.3.1 Tocolysis therapy

When preterm labour is diagnosed in twin pregnancies, its management should be done taking in account several factors such as maternal and fetal risks. The use of tocolytics for the treatment of preterm labour has not been shown to decrease the incidence of delivery within 7 days of treatment or perinatal death (Anotayanonth et al, 2004). The lack of proven efficacy, the high incidence of side-effects with some drugs such as adrenergic receptors agonists should be taken in account in the tocolysis guidelines for multiple gestations (ACOG, 2004). In Europe, atosiban and nifedipine seem to have the best balance between efficiency and side-effects profile. The role of progesterone should still be evaluated in randomized controlled trials (Dodd et al, 2008).

In contrast to tocolytics, the use of antenatal corticosteroids has been shown to decrease the incidence of neonatal death and others neonatal complications (respiratory distress syndrome, intraventricular hemorrhage, necrotizing enterocolitis) (Roberts et al, 2006). Tocolytic drugs should then aim to allow the pregnant patient transfer to a tertiary referral center or to ensure a proper antenatal corticosteroids course administration.

6.3.2 Cerclage

Another approach to decrease premature births could be to reinforce the cervix with a cerclage. The use of history-indicated (prophylactic) cerclage for twins gestation in a randomized trial did not decrease the rate of prematurity significantly (45% with cerclage vs. 48% without suture) or neonatal mortality (18% vs. 15% for suture vs. no suture, respectively) (Dor et al, 1982). More important, when cerclage was used in asymptomatic woman with twin gestations and short cervical length on transvaginal ultrasound examination, it significantly increased the risk of delivery at < 35 weeks of gestation (Berghella et al, 2005). Thus, cerclage of asymptomatic short cervical length should be avoided for twin gestations. Treatments that prevent preterm birth in singleton pregnancies, such as progesterone and cervical cerclage appear to be ineffective in multiple pregnancies (Stock et al, 2010).

6.4 Delayed twin delivery

One of the most common and serious complications of multiple gestations is preterm delivery. In some cases, preterm delivery of one fetus may occur without spontaneous delivery of the remaining fetus. This unique event raises the possibility of prolonging a pregnancy to a more advanced gestational age before delivery of the remaining fetus. The benefits of a delayed delivery can lead to a significant decrease in neonatal morbidity and mortality. During critical gestational ages, delayed delivery can also change the risk of delivering a periviable baby with severe morbidity related to prematurity instead of delivering a previable fetus. Attempts to delay delivery should only be undertaken in the absence of any maternal or fetal indications for delivery. Unfavorable conditions for delayed interval delivery are: monochorionic placentation, evidence of intrauterine infection, rupture of membranes of the retained fetus, placental abruption and fetal abnormalities. The gestational age at the time of delivery of the first fetus should be at least 16 to 18 weeks before prolonged interval delivery is considered (Farkouh et al, 2000). The conservative management of triplet pregnancy after delivery of one fetus is a feasible and reasonable approach and is not associated with significantly increased fetal-maternal morbidity (Biard et al, 2000). At the present time, the optimal management of a delayed delivery is not known, but immediate cerclage, broad-spectrum antibiotics, tocolysis and steroids for fetal lung maturity are a reasonable strategy (Graham et al, 2005).

7. Intrapartum prevention of multiple pregnancy related to perinatal mortality

7.1 Choice of delivery for uncomplicated twins

There is a general consensus that vaginal delivery for twins is safe when both are in vertex presentation, whereas planned caesarean section is typically indicated for breech presentation of the first twin.

A systematic review (Rossi et al, 2011) suggests that an attempt at vaginal delivery should be considered in twin pregnancies without inter-twin birth weight discordance (of more than 20%) and very low birth weight (< 1500g). Current literature shows that in twins with vertex/vertex presentation, vaginal delivery is safer than caesarean section for the first twin, and no differences are observed for the second twin after vaginal or caesarean section. In pregnancies with vertex presentation of the first twin and non-vertex presentation of the second twin, women should be counselled that trial of labour is a safe option in the absence of risk factors that may increase the risk of a caesarean delivery of the second twin after vaginal delivery of the first twin.

It is desirable for women with a twin pregnancy to have epidural analgesia. Vaginal delivery should be performed by an obstetrician with experience in the vaginal delivery of twins (Vayssière et al, 2007).

There is no reason to recommended one type of delivery rather than another in twin pregnancies, regardless of gestational age at birth. For both vertex/vertex and vertex/non-vertex presentations, morbidity and mortality are similar for vaginal and caesarean deliveries of twin gestations at or beyond 30 weeks of gestation and with birth weight twin greater than 1500 g (Peaceman et al, 2009).

At the present time, an international randomised controlled trial - the Twin Birth Study, coordinated by the University of Toronto - is underway. This study aims to provide more reliable information as to the optimal mode of delivery of uncomplicated twins. This study is in progress and the first results will be available in May 2012.

7.2 Delivery of the second twin

The systematic review (Rossi et al, 2011) describes a mild reduction of neonatal death occurred after vaginal delivery in both vertex and non-vertex presentation of the second twin as compared with caesarean section.

Active management of the delivery of the second twin is recommended to reduce the interval between the births of the two twins, because this interval is associated with:

- Progressive degradation of neonatal acid-base indicators,
- Increase in the number of caesareans for the second twin,
- Neonatal morbidity of the second twin,
- Obstetrical complications including placental abruption, umbilical cord prolapse, uterine atony and cervical spasm.

In the case of non-vertex presentation, total breech extraction, preceded by internal version manoeuvres if the twin's position is transverse, is associated with the lowest caesarean rates for second twins. In these situations, external cephalic version may be harmful. In the case of a high and not yet engaged cephalic presentation and if team is appropriately trained, version by internal manoeuvres followed by total breech extraction is to be preferred to a combination of resumption of pushing, oxytocin perfusion, and artificial rupture of the membranes, because the former strategy appears to be associated with fewer caesareans for the second twin. In the case of an engaged cephalic presentation, management should involve resumption of pushing, oxytocin perfusion, and artificial rupture of the membranes.

Obstetric manoeuvres on the second twin should be practised as first-line treatment with intact membranes (Vayssière et al, 2011).

A large dataset of twin deliveries (Peaceman et al, 2009) supports the safety of breech extraction for the non-vertex second twin, in contrast to studies of singleton breech vaginal deliveries, with their higher reported rates of morbidity and head entrapment. Perhaps this is because the larger twin usually delivers first, diminishing the chances that the cervix will be insufficiently dilated for the subsequent breech delivery.

7.3 Delivery of monochorionic pregnancies

7.3.1 Delivery of monochorionic diamniotic twins

A large cohort of monochorionic twin pregnancies without TTTS reported a risk of fetal death after 32 weeks of 5 in 1000 births and an incidence of perinatal mortality in term monochorionic twins of 7 per 1000 infants (Hack et al, 2011). This is three-fold higher than in term singletons and term dichorionic twin pregnancies. Unfortunately, current antenatal surveillance (i.e. fetal heart monitoring, fetal ultrasound and Doppler studies) fails to predict and prevent intrauterine fetal death. The increased risk of (unexpected) intrauterine fetal death (even at term), with subsequent consequences for the surviving twin (possible co-twin death or brain damage), and the failure to predict and prevent all cases of excess intrauterine fetal death by current antenatal care raise the question as to when to deliver monochorionic twins. Offering planned delivery between 36 and 37 weeks seems therefore to be the best consensus by preventing term mortality and avoiding the risk of neonatal respiratory disorders that is linked to preterm delivery (Escobar et al, 2006).

The contribution of mode of delivery to the increased perinatal mortality in monochorionic twins is not clear and there is no consensus regarding the optimal mode of delivery.

The monochorionic twins are more likely to have intrapartum complications as acute TTTS during labour. These complications may necessitate emergency caesarean delivery. Such complications could be prevented by offering planned caesarean section to all monochorionic twin pregnancies, as has been suggested in the literature (Smith et al, 2005). However, these benefits should be weighed against the risks of neonatal respiratory morbidity in infants delivered by planned caesarean section and maternal complications from the caesarean section.

There is a need for randomised data to determine the best strategy with respect to when and how to deliver the monochorionic twins.

7.3.2 Delivery of monochorionic monoamniotic twins

The timing of delivery in monoamniotic pregnancies is a balance between the risk of preterm birth and the risk of intrauterine death at a given gestation. The basis for timed elective delivery is to prevent cord-related deaths. Recent publication advocates delivery at 32-34 weeks gestation after corticosteroid maturation, when perinatal mortality rates in most neonatal intensive care units at gestations of 34 weeks are very low.

The majority of units use caesarean birth as the preferred delivery mode for monoamniotic twins. Caesarean delivery offers more control over complex events such as umbilical cord entanglement with difficulty in delivery of second twin (Dickinson et al, 2005).

8. Conclusion

Twins and higher-order multiple pregnancies are well known to carry a higher risk of adverse outcomes compared with singletons. Multiple pregnancies present numerous challenges for the obstetrician from conception onwards, until the timing and mode of delivery. The stillbirth rate in twins is four times and neonatal mortality is five to seven higher than in singletons (Anthony et al, 2009). The main cause of mortality is preterm birth and its short and long-term sequelae. Monochorionicity adverse effects, aneuploidy, congenital malformations, growth restriction, single fetal demise and delivery related problems are additional factors for increased perinatal mortality and should be diagnosed as soon as possible. A systematic ultrasound careful exam should be offered to these pregnancies (Hubinont et al, 2010). This chapter illustrates most of the complications of multiple pregnancies and the prevention of perinatal mortality. The higher risks have been shown in monochorionic pregnancies. All of these high-risk pregnancies require careful consideration with regard to the management of their specific complications in a maternal-fetal medicine center.

9. References

Allen V, Windrim R, Barrett J, Ohlsson A. Management of monoamniotic twin pregnancies: a case series and systematic review of the literature. *BJOG* 2001;108:931-936.

American College of Obstetricians and Gynecologists; Society of Maternal-Fetal Medicine. Multiple gestation: complicated twin, triplet, and higher-order multifetal pregnancy. Washington, DC: The College; 2004.

Ananth CV, Joseph KS, Smulian JC. Trends in twin neonatal mortality rates in the United States, 1989 through 1999: influence of birth registration and obstetric intervention. *Am J Obstet Gynecol* 2004;190:1313-1321.

Anotayanonth S, Subhedar NV, Garner P, Neilson JP, Harigopal S. Betamimetics for inhibiting preterm labour. *Cochrane Database Syst Rev* 2004;4:CD004352.

Anthony S, Jacobusse GW, van der Pal-de Bruin KM, Buitendijk S, Zeitlin J. Do differences in maternal age, parity and multiple births explain variations in fetal and neonatal mortality rates in Europe? - results from the EURO-PERISTAT project. *Paediatr Perin Epidemiol* 2009;23:292-300.

Arabin L, Laurini RN, van Eyck J. Early prenatal diagnosis of cord entanglement in monoamniotic multiple pregnancies. *Ultrasound Obstet Gynecol* 1999;13:140-142.

Bajoria R, Kingdom J. The case for routine determination of chorionicity and zygosity in multiple pregnancy. *Prenat Diagn* 1997;17:1207-25.

Barrea C, Hornberger L, Alkazaleh F, et al. Impact of selective laser ablation of placental anastomoses on the cardiovascular pathology of the recipient twin in severe twin-twin transfusion syndrome. *Am J Obstet Gynecol* 2006;195:1388-1395.

Barrett JFR. Delivery of the term twin. *Best Pract Res Clin Obstet Gynaecol* 2004;18(4):625-630.

Bahtiyar MO, Dulay AT, Weeks BP, Friedman AH, Copel JA. Prevalence of congenital heart defects in monochorionic/diamniotic twin gestations. A systematic literature review. *J Ultrasound Med* 2007;26:1491-1498.

Benirschke K. Intrauterine death of a twin: mechanisms, implications for surviving twin, and placenta pathology. *Semin Diagn Pathol* 1993;10:222-31.

Berghella V, Odibo A, To M, Rust O, Althuisius S. Cerclage for short cervix on ultrasound meta-analysis of trials using individual patient-level data. *Obstet Gynecol* 2005;106:181-9.

Bhide A, Sankaran S, Sairam S, Papageorghiou A, Thilaganathan B. Relationship of intertwine crown-rump length discrepancy to chorionicity, fetal demise and birth-weight discordance. *Ultrasound Obstet Gynecol* 2009;34:131-135.

Biard JM, Bernard P, Thomas K, Hubinont C. Conservative management of triplet pregnancy after delivery of one fetus. *Twin Res* 2000;3(2):71-5.

Black M, Bhattacharya S. Epidemiology of multiple pregnancy and the effect of assisted conception. *Semin Fetal Neonatal Med* 2010;15(6):306-12.

Blondel B, Kaminski M. L'augmentation des naissances multiples et ses conséquences en santé périnatale. *J Gynecol Obstet Biol Reprod* 2002;31:725-740.

Chang YL, Chang SD, Chao AS, et al. Clinical outcome and placental territory ratio of monochorionic twin pregnancies and selective intrauterine growth restriction with different types of umbilical artery Doppler. *Prenat Diagn* 2009;29:253-256.

Chalouhi GE, Essaoui M, Stirnemann J, Quibel T, Deloison B, Salomon L, Ville Y. Laser therapy for twin-to-twin transfusion syndrome (TTTS). *Prenat Diagn* 2011;31:637-646.

Chauhan S, Scardo J, Hayes E, Abuhamad A, Berghella V. Twins: prevalence, problems, and preterm births. *Am J Obstet Gynecol* 2010;203(4):305-315.

Chelli D, Methni A, Boudaya F, et al. Grossesse gémellaire avec mort foetale in utero d'un jumeau: étiologies, prise en charge et pronostic. *J Gynecol Biol Reprod* 2009;38:580-587.

Cheng PJ, Huang SY, Shaw SW, et al. Difference in nuchal translucency between monozygotic and dizygotic spontaneously conceived twins. *Prenat Diagn* 2010;30:247-250.

Cheng PJ, Shaw SW, Shih JC, Soong YK. Monozygotic twins discordant for monosomy 21detected by first-trimester nuchal translucency thickness. *Obstet Gynecol* 2006;107:538-541.

Cordero L, Franco A, Joy SD, O'Shaughnessy RW. Monochorionic diamniotic infants without twin-to-twin transfusion syndrome. *J Perinatol* 2005;25:753-758.

Cordero L, Franco A, Joy SD. Monochorionic monoamniotic twins: neonatal outcome. *J Perinatol* 2006;26:170-175.

De Mouzon J, Lancaster P, Nygren KG, et al. World collaborative report on assisted reproductive technology, 2002. *Hum Reprod* 2009;1:1-11.

Dias T, Mahsud-Dornan S, Bhide A, Papageorghiou A, Thilaganathan B. Cord entanglement and perinatal outcome in monoamniotic twin pregnancies. *Ultrasound Obstet Gynecol* 2010;35:201-204.

Dias T, Mahsud-Dornan S, Thilaganathan B, Papageorhiou A, Bhide A. First-trimester ultrasound dating of twin pregnancy: are singleton charts reliable? *BJOG* 2010;117:979-984.

Dickinson J. Monoamniotic twin pregnancy: a review of contemporary practice. *Aust N Z J Obstet Gynecol* 2005;45:474-478.

Dodd JM, Flenady VJ, Cincotta R, Crowther CA. Progesterone for the prevention of preterm birth a systematic review. *Obstet Gynecol* 2008;112:127-34.

Dor J, Shalev J, Mashiach S, et al. Elective cervical suture of twin pregnancies diagnosed ultrasonically in the first trimester following induced ovulation. *Gynecol Obstet Invest* 1982;13:55-60.

Edlow A, Reiss R, Benson C, Gerrol P, Wilkins-Haug L. Monochorionic diamniotic twin gestations discordant for markedly enlarged nuchal translucency. *Prenat Diagn* 2011;31:299-306.

Elliott JP, Urig MA, Clewell WH. Aggressive therapeutic amniocentesis for the treatment of twin-twin transfusion syndrome. *Obstet Gynecol* 1991;77:537-40.

Escobar GJ, Clark RH, Greene JD. Short-term outcomes of infants born at 35 and 36 weeks gestation: we need to ask more questions. *Semin Perinatol* 2006;30:28-33.

Evans MI, Kaufman MI, Urban AJ, Britt DW, Fletcher JC. Fetal reduction from twins to a singleton: a reasonable consideration? *Obstet Gynecol* 2004;104:102-109.

Evans MI, Ciorica D, Britt DW, Fletcher JC. Update on selective reduction. *Prenat Diagn* 2005;25:807-813.

Ezra Y, Shveiky D, OphirE, Nadjari M, Eisenberg VH, Samueloff A, Rojansky N. Intensive management and early delivery reduce antenatal mortality in monoamniotic twin pregnancies. *Acta Obstet Gynecol Scand* 2005;84:432-435.

Farkouh LJ, Sabin ED, Heyborn KD, et al. Delayed-interval delivery: Extended series from a single maternal-fetal medicine practice. *Am J Obstet Gynecol* 2000;183:1499-1503.

Fichera A, Lanna M, Fratelli N, Rustico M, Frusca T. Twin-to-twin transfusion syndrome presenting at early stages: is there still a possible role for amnioreduction? *Prenat Diagn* 2010;30:144-8.

Fichera A, Zambolo C, Accorsi P, et al. Perinatal outcome and neurological follow-up of the co-twins in twin pregnancies complicated by single intrauterine death. *Eur J Obstet Gynecol Reprod Biol* 2009 Nov;147(1):37-40.

Fisk NM, Borrell A, Hubinont C, Tannirandorn Y, Nicolini U, Rodeck CH. Fetofetal transfusion syndrome : do the neonatal criteria apply in utero ? *Arch Dis Child* 1990,65 :657-661.

Glinianaia SV, Obeysekera MA, Sturgiss S, Bell R. Stillbirth and neonatal mortality in monochorionic and dichorionic twins : a population-based study. *Hum Reprod* 2011;0 :1-9.

Goldman JC, D'Alton ME. Growth abnormalities and multiple gestations. *Semin Perinatol* 2008;32 :206-212.

Goncé A, Borrell A, Meler E, et al. Prevalence and perinatal outcome of dichorionic and monochorionic twins with nuchal translucency above the 99th percentile and normal karyotype. *Ultrasound Obstet Gynecol* 2010;35 :14-18.

Graham G, Gaddipati S. Diagnosis and management of obstetrical complications unique to multiple gestations. *Semin Perinatol* 2005;29 :282-295.

Gratacos E, Lewi L, Carreras E, et al. Incidence and characteristics of umbilical artery intermittent absent and/or reversed end-diastolic flow in complicated and uncomplicated monochorionic twin pregnancies. *Ultrasound Obstet Gynecol* 2004;23 :456-60.

Gratacos E, Lewi L, Munoz B, et al. A classification system for selective intrauterine growth restriction in monochorionic pregnancies according to umbilical artery Doppler flow in the smaller twin. *Ultrasound Obstet Gynecol* 2007;30:28-34.

Gucciardo L, Lewi L, Vaast P, et al. Twin anemia polycythemia sequence from a prenatal perspective. *Prenat Diagn* 2010;30:438-442.

Hack K, Derks J, Elias S, et al. Increased perinatal mortality and morbidity in monochorionic versus dichorionic twin pregnancies: clinical implications of a large Dutch cohort study. *BJOG* 2008;115:58-67.

Hack K, Derks J, Schaap A, Lopriore E, Elias S, Arabin B, Eggink A, Sollie K, Mol B, Duvekot H, Willekes C, Go A, Koopman-Esseboom C, Vandenbussche F, Visser G. Perinatal outcome of monoamniotic twin pregnancies. *Obstet Gynecol* 2009;113:353-360.

Hack K, Derks J, Elias S, et al. Perinatal mortality and mode of delivery in monochorionic diamniotic twin pregnancies > 32 weeks of gestation: a multicentre retrospective cohort study. *BJOG* 2011;DOI:10.1111/j.1471-0528.2011.02955.x.

Haverkamp F, Lex C, Hanisch C, Fahnenstich H, Zerres K. Neurodevelopmental risks in twin-to-twin transfusion syndrome: preliminary findings. *Eur J Paediatr Neurol* 2001;5:21-27.

Hendrix NW, Chauhan SP. Sonographic examination of twins. From first trimester to delivery of second fetus. *Obstet Gynecol Clin North Am* 1998;25:609-621.

Herbst A, Källén K. Influence of mode of delivery on neonatal mortality in the second twin, at and before term. *BJOG* 2008;115;1512-1517.

Hillman SC, Morris RK, Kilby MD. Single twin demise: consequence for survivors. *Semin Fetal Neonatal Med* 2010;15:319-326.

Hubinont C, Santolaya-Forgas J. A systematic approach to first-trimester ultrasound assessment of twins. *Am J Perinatol* 2010;27:595-598.

Hubinont C, Bernard P, Pirot N, Biard JM, Donnez J. Twin-to-twin transfusion syndrome: treatment by amniodrainage and septostomy. *Eur J Obstet Gynecol Reprod Biol* 2000;92(1):141-144.

Hubinont C, Bernard P, Mwebesa W, Magritte JP, Donnez J. Nd:YAG laser and needle disruption of the interfetal septum: A possible therapy in severe twin-to-twin transfusion syndrome. *J Gynecol Surg* 1996;12:183-9.

Hubinont C, Kollman P, Malvaux V, Donnez J, Bernard P. First-trimester diagnosis of conjoined twins. *Fetal Diagn Ther* 1997;12(3):185-7.

Hubinont C, Pratola D, Rothschild E, Rodesch F, Schwers J. Dicephalus: unusual case of conjoined twins and its prepartum diagnosis. *Am J Obstet Gynecol* 1984;149(6):693-4.

Ishii K, Murakoshi T, Takahashi Y, et al. Perinatal outcome of monochorionic twins with selective intrauterine growth restriction and different types of umbilical artery Doppler under expectant management. *Fetal Diagn Ther* 2009;26:157-61.

Ishii K, Murakoshi T, Hayashi S, et al. Ultrasound predictors of mortality in monochorionic twins with selective intrauterine growth restriction. *Ultrasound Obstet Gynecol* 2011;37:22-26.

Kagan K, Gazzoni A, Sepulveda-Gonzalez G, Sotiriadis A, Nicolaides K. Discordance in nuchal translucency thickness in the prediction of severe twin-to-twin transfusion syndrome. *Ultrasound Obstet Gynecol* 2007;29:527-532.

Kilby MD, Govind A, O'Brien PM. Outcome of twin pregnancies complicated by a single intrauterine death: a comparison with viable twin pregnancies. *Obstet Gynecol* 1994;84:107-9.

Lewi L, Cannie M, Blickstein I, Jani J, Huber A, Hecher K, Dymarkowski S, Gratacos E, Lewi P, Deprest J. Placental sharing, birthweight discordance, and vascular anastomoses in monochorionic diamniotic twin placentas. *Am J Obstet Gynecol* 2007;197:587.e1-587.e8.

Lewi L, Lewi P, Diemert A, Jani J, Gucciardo L, Van Mieghem T, Doné E, Gratacos E, Huber A, Hecher K, Deprest J. The role of ultrasound examination in the first trimester and at 16 weeks'gestation to predict fetal complications in monochorionic diamniotic twin pregnancies. *Am J Obstet Gynecol* 2008.199:493.e1-493.e7.

Lewi L, Jani J, Blickstein I, Huber A, Gucciardo L, Van Mieghem T, Doné E, Boes AS, Hecher K, Gratacos E, Lewi P, Deprest J. The outcome of monochorionic diamniotic twin gestations in the era of invasive fetal therapy: a prospective cohort study. *Am J Obstet Gynecol* 2008;199:514.e1-514.e8.

Lewi L, Gucciardo L, Huber A, et al. Clinical outcome and placental characteristics of monochorionic diamniotic twin pairs with early- and late-onset discordant growth. *Am J Obstet Gynecol* 2008;199:511.e1-7.

Lewi L, Gucciardo L, Van Mieghem T, De Koninck Ph, Beck V, Medek H, Van Schoubroeck D, Devlieger R, De Catte L, Deprest J. Monochorionic diamniotic twin pregnancies: natural history and risk stratification. *Fetal Diagn Ther* 2010;27:121-133.

Lewi L, Valencia C, Gonzalez E, Deprest J, Nicolaides K. The outcome of twin reversed arterial perfusion sequence diagnosed in the first trimester. *Am J Obstet Gynecol* 2010;203:213.e1-4.

Livingston JC, Lim FY, Mason J, Crombleholme M. Intrafetal radiofrequency ablation for twin reversed arterial perfusion (TRAP): a single-center experience. *Am J Obstet Gynecol* 2007;197:399.e1-399.e3.

Lopriore E, Middeldorp JM, Oepkes D, Kanhai HH, Walther FJ, Vandenbussche FP. Twin anemia-polycythemia sequence in two monochorionic twin pairs without oligo-polyhydramnios sequence. *Placenta* 2007;28:47-51.

Manning N, Archer N. A study to determine the incidence of structural congenital heart disease in monochorionic twins. *Prenat Diagn* 2006;26:1062-1064.

Maschke C, Diemert A, Hecher K, Bartmann P. Long-term outcome after intrauterine laser treatment for twin-twin transfusion syndrome. *Prenat Diagn* 2011;31:647-653.

Mastroiacovo P, Castilla EE, Arpino C, Botting B, Cocchi G, Goujard J, Marinacci C, Merlob P, Metneki J, Mutchinick O, Ritvanen A, Rosano A. Congenital malformations in twins: an international study. *Am J Med Genet* 1999;83:117-124.

Moore TR, Gale S, Benirschke K. Perinatal outcome of forty-nine pregnancies complicated by acardiac twinning. *Am J Obstet Gynecol* 1990;163:907-12.

Myrianthopoulos NC. Congenital malformations: the contribution of twin studies. *Birth Defects Orig Artic Ser* 1978;14:151-165.

Nicolini U, Poblete A. Single intrauterine death in monochorionic twin pregnancies. *Ultrasound Obstet Gynecol* 1999;14(5):297-301.

O'Donoghue K, Rutheford MA, Engineer N, Wimalasundera RC, Cowan FM, Fisk NM. Transfusional fetal complications after single intrauterine death in monochorionic multiple pregnancy are reduced but not prevented by vascular occlusion. *BJOG* 2009;116:804-812.

Ong SS, Zamora J, Khan KH, Kilby MD. Prognosis for the co-twin following single-twin death: a systematic review. *BJOG* 2006;113(9):992-8.

Pasquini L, Wimalasundera RC, Fichera A, Barigye O, Chapell L, Fisk NM. High perinatal survival in monoamniotic twins managed by prophylactic sulindac, intensive ultrasound surveillance, and Cesarean delivery at 32 weeks'gestation. *Ultrasound Obstet Gynecol* 2006;28:681-687.

Peaceman AM, Kuo L, Feinglass J. Infant morbidity and mortality associated with vaginal delivery in twin gestations. *Am J Obstet Gynecol* 2009;200:462.e1-462.e6.

Quintero R, Morales W, Allen M, Bornick P, Johnson P, Kruger M. Staging of twin-twin transfusion syndrome. *J Perinatol* 1999;19:550-5.

Roberts D, Dalziel S. Antenatal corticosteroids for accelerating fetal lung maturation for women at risk of preterm birth. *Cochrane Database Syst Rev* 2006;3:CD004454.

Robyr R, Lewi L, Salomon LJ, Yamamoto M, Bernard JP, Deprest J, Ville Y. Prevalence and management of late fetal complications following successful selective laser coagulation of chorionic plate anastomoses in twin-to-twin transfusion syndrome. *Am J Obstet Gynecol* 2006;194:796-803.

Rossi AC, Mullin PM, Chmait RH. Neonatal outcomes of twins according to birth order, presentation and mode of delivery: a systematic review and meta-analysis. *BJOG* 2011;118:523-532.

Rychik J, Tian Z, Bebbington M, et al. The twin-twin transfusion syndrome: spectrum of cardiovascular abnormality and development of a cardiovascular score to assess severity of disease. *Am J Obstet Gynecol* 2007;197:392.e1-8.

Shah AD, Border WL, Crombleholme TM, Michelfelder EC. Initial fetal cardiovascular profile score predicts recipient twin outcome in twin-twin transfusion syndrome. *J Am Soc Echocardiogr* 2008;21:1105-1108.

Sau AK, Langford K, Elliot C, Su LL, Maxwell DJ. Monoamniotic twins: what should be the optimal antenatal management? *Twin Res* 2003.6:270-274.

Sebire NJ, Souka A, Skentou, H, Geerts L, Nicolaides KH. Early prediction of severe twin-to-twin transfusion syndrome. *Hum Reprod* 2000;15:2008-2010.

Senat MV, Deprest J, Boulvain M, Paupe A, Winer N, Ville Y. Endoscopic laser surgery versus serial amnioreduction for severe twin-to-twin transfusion syndrome. *N Engl J Med* 2004;351(2):136-44.

Senat MV, Quarello E, Levaillant JM, Buonumano A, Boulvain M, Frydman R. Determining chorionicity in twin gestations: three-dimensional (3D) multiplanar sonographic measurement of intra-amniotic membrane thickness. *Ultrasound Obstet Gynecol* 2006;28:665-669.

Sepulveda W, Sebire NJ, Hughes K, Kalogeropoulos A, Nicolaides KH. Evolution of the lambda or twin-chorionic peak sign in dichorionic twin pregnancies. *Obstet Gynecol* 1997;89(3):439-441.

Sepulveda W, Wong A, Casasbuenas A. Nuchal translucency and nasal bone in first-trimester ultrasound screening for aneuploidy in multiple pregnancies. *Ultrasound Obstet Gynecol* 2009;33:152-156.

Spencer K, Kagan KO, Nicolaides KH. Screening for trisomy 21 in twin pregnancies in the first trimester: an update of the impact of chorionicity on maternal serum markers. *Prenat Diagn* 2008;28:49-52.

Smith GC, Shah I, White IR, Pell JP, Dobbie R. Mode of delivery and the risk of delivery-related perinatal death among twins at term: a retrospective cohort study of 8073 births. *BJOG* 2005;112:1139-44.

Sperling L, Kill C, Larsen L et al. Detection of chromosomal abnormalities, congenital abnormalities and transfusion syndrome in twins. *Ultrasound Obstet Gynecol* 2007;29:517-526.

Stirnemann JJ, Mougeot M, Proulx F, et al. Profiling fetal cardiac function in twin-twin transfusion syndrome. *Ultrasound Obstet Gynecol* 2010a;35:19-27.

Stirnemann JJ, Nasr B, Proulx F, Essaoui M, Ville Y. Evaluation of the CHOP cardiovascular score as a prognostic predictor of outcome in twin-twin transfusion syndrome after laser coagulation of placental vessels in a prospective cohort. *Ultrasound Obstet Gynecol* 2010b;36:52-57.

Stock S, Norman J. Preterm and term labour in multiple pregnancies. *Semin Fetal Neonatal Med* 2010;15:336-341.

Tandberg A, Melve K, Nordtveit T, et al. Maternal birth characteristics and perinatal mortality in twin offspring. An intergenerational population-based study in Norway, 1967-2008. *BJOG* 2011;118:698-705.

Valsky D, Eixarch E, Martinez J, Crispi F, Gratacos E. Selective intrauterine growth restriction in monochorionic twins: pathophysiology, diagnostic approach and management dilemmas. *Semin Fetal Neonatal Med* 2010;15:342-348.

Valsky D, Eixarch E, Martinez J, Gratacos E. Selective intrauterine growth restriction in monochorionic diamniotic twin pregnancies. *Prenat Diagn* 2010;30:719-726.

Vanderheyden TM, Fichera A, Pasquini L, et al. Increased latency of absent end-diastolic flow in the umbilical artery of monochorionic twin fetuses. *Ultrasound Obstet Gynecol* 2005;26:44-9.

Vayssière Ch, Benoist G, Blondel B, Deruelle Ph, Favre R, et al. Twin pregnancies: guidelines for clinical practice from the French College of Gynaecologists and Obstetricians (CNGOF). *Eur J Obstet Gynecol Reprod Biol* 2011;156:12-17.

Vendittelli F, Accoceberry M, Savary D, et al. Quelle voie d'accouchement pour les jumeaux? *J Gynecol Obstet Biol Reprod* 2009;38:S104-S113.

Wan JJ, Schrimmer D, Taché V, Quinn K, Lacoursiere Y, James G, Benirschke K, Pretorius DH. Current practices in determining amnionicity and chorionicity in multiple gestations. *Prenat Diagn* 2011;31:125-130.

Wimalasundera RC, Trew G, Fisk NM. Reducing the incidence of twins and triplets. Best Pract Res Clin Obstet Gynaecol *2003*;17:309-329.

Wimalasundera RC. Selective reduction and termination of multiple pregnancies. *Semin Fetal Neonatal Med* 2010;15(6):327-35.

Zoppi MA. Nuchal translucency screening in monochorionic twin pregnancies. *Ultrasound Obstet Gynecol* 2009;34:491-493.

6

Helicopter Transportation for Perinatal and Maternal Emergency Care in Japan

Ryuzo Higuchi and Sawako Minami
Divisions of NICU and Obstetrics,
Department of Perinatal Medicine,
Wakayama Medical University
Japan

1. Introduction

The number of obstetric and pediatric doctors has been the most insufficient in all the fields of clinical medicine even in the age of decreasing birthrate in Japan. Obstetric departments in local hospitals and private obstetric clinics have been closed and reorganized especially in the sparsely populated areas during late 10 years. The perinatal transportation system becomes more critical than ever before to maintain the quality of perinatal medicine.

The Helicopter Emergency Medical Service was started in Japan in 2001 after the civil aeronautic law was partly amended to allow the service. The so-called "doctor-helicopter law" was then enacted in 2007 to promote introduction of the Helicopter Emergency Medical Service nationwide based on governmental funding. As of June 2011, 27 helicopters are in emergency medical service in the field of emergency medicine (Japanese Society for Aeromedical Services, 2011). Since Japan is an island country and has many isolated islands, helicopters have sporadically been involved in the maternal or neonatal transportations. However, there seems to be no other hospitals like Wakayama Medical University Hospital where a helicopter routinely has taken part in the maternal and neonatal transportation that obstetric and pediatric doctors are involved in, respectively.

The objective is to study the effectiveness of helicopter transport in the perinatal medicine.

2. Methods

2.1 Helicopter emergency medical service at wakayama medical university hospital

In January 2003, Wakayama Medical University Hospital became the 7th hospital in Japan to introduce a helicopter for Emergency Medical Service. The helicopter, a Eurocopter EC135Pi, is based at the rooftop of the 13-story university hospital, and the helicopter administration office where communication center is, and medical and flight crews are standing by is on the 13th floor. Emergency room and perinatal medical center are on the first and 6th floors of the same building, respectively. The helicopter was installed with a respirator, a cardiorespiratory monitor, a portable echo, and an automated external defibrillator. The hospital is located in northwest Wakayama prefecture. The coverage area is the whole of Wakayama prefecture (4,726.12 km^2), the southern part of Nara prefecture (1,727.52 km^2), and the southern part of Mie prefecture (991.74 km^2). The flying time is 30 minutes for 100 km. Service hours are 8:00 am to 5:00 pm (6:00 pm in summer) and the crew comprises a pilot, co-pilot, emergency medical doctor, and emergency medical nurse. The flight frequency is currently 390/year (0-5/day).

2.2 Modifications of the helicopter emergency medical service for perinatal transfer

Wakayama Medical University Perinatal Medical Center, the only one tertiary perinatal medical center in Wakayama prefecture (Section on Transport Medicine American Academy of Pediatrics, 2007), was equipped with a vehicle installed with a neonatal respirator, two incubators, and two cardiorespiratory monitors for neonatal ground transfer in 2000. Use of the helicopter emergency medical service for perinatal and maternal medical transport began in June 2003 and some modifications were needed in order to provide these services. Perinatal medical transport was for high-risk pregnant women or sick neonates, and basically limited to inter-facility transport. The crew is comprised of the 4 personnel described above, plus a neonatal intensive care doctor (NICU) for neonatal transport or an obstetric doctor for maternal transport. The NICU or obstetrics department receive the request for helicopter transport from a local medical facility and ask the helicopter administration office to set up the rendezvous point and time with the local ambulance office, which then transfer the patient from the local medical facility to the rendezvous point. The NICU doctor on departure loads a neonatal transport incubator into the helicopter. The coverage area include the whole of Wakayama prefecture and the southern part of Mie prefecture from which it takes more than 3 hours to transport a patient to the perinatal center overland. The frequency of neonatal and maternal transports has been 4-11/year each since the services were introduced.

Statistical data from 2003 indicated that south Wakayama (SW) comprised 50.4% of the area, 19.6% of the population, and 20.7% of the live births in Wakayama Prefecture; and south Mie (SM) comprised 17.2% of the area, 4.7% of the population, and 3.4% of the live births in Mie Prefecture (Fig. 1)

Perinatal helicopter transportation was started in June 2003, and therefore maternal and child health statistics were compared for the three years before (2000-2002) and after (2004-2006) this year, (Department of Health and Welfare, Mie Prefecture; Department of Health and Welfare, Wakayama Prefecture; & Ministry of Health, Labor, and Welfare) using a χ-square test and Fisher's exact test. The neonatal mortality rate was defined as number of deaths at < 28 days after birth in three years / number of live births in three years × 1,000 - and the perinatal mortality rate as perinatal deaths (fetal deaths after 22 weeks of pregnancy + early neonatal deaths) in three years / total births (live births + fetal deaths after 22 weeks of pregnancy) in three years× 1,000. The fetal death rate was defined as fetal deaths in three years / total births in three years × 1,000 (Mothers' & Children's Health & Welfare Association, 2006).

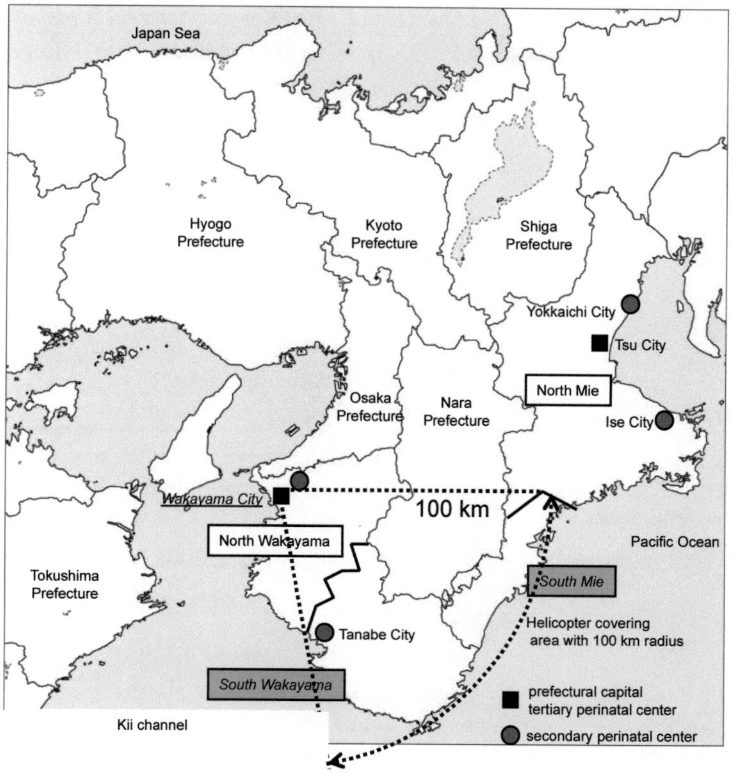

Fig. 1. Tanabe City is the central part of Wakayama prefecture. South Wakayama (SW) is Tanabe City and south of it, and north Wakayama (NW) is north of it. Perinatal Helicopter Medical Service covers area within the 100 km radius, mainly SW and south Mie (SM).

3. Results

3.1 The result of the perinatal and maternal emergency helicopter transport from June 2003 to Dec 2010 is presented

3.1.1 Neonatal helicopter transportation

There were 51 cases of neonatal transfer by helicopter (6.8 cases/year), one of which was a pair of twins, during the time period from June 2003 to December 2010. The reasons of transport were critical congenital cardiac disease (n=19), neonatal asphyxia (n=12), congenital digestive tract anomaly (n=7), low birth weight (n=5, including 3 extremely low birth weight (ELBW) infants), neonatal jaundice (n=4), respiratory distress (n=3), post-hemorrhagic hydrocephalus (n=1), and neonatal vomiting (n=1) (Table 1).

The referring facilities were located in north Wakayama (NW) (n=17) and south Wakayama (SW) (n=34) based on division of the prefecture into north and south with respect to the location of Tanabe City, which is in central Wakayama (Fig. 2). The average time from request of helicopter transport by a local hospital until take-off and return to site 13R of the university hospital was 23 ± 23 min and 1 hr, 23 ± 33 min (mean ± 1S.D), respectively.

Reasons for neonatal transports	*No.(%)*	*Reasons for maternal transports*	*No.(%)*
Critical congenital cardiac disease	19 (37.3)	Threatened premeture delivery	25(46.3)
Neonatal asphyxia	12(23.5)	Preterm PROM	13(24.1)
Congenital digestive tract anomaly	7(13.7)	Pregnancy induced hypertension	4(7.4)
Low birth weight (ELBW)	4*(7.8))	Threatened abortion	3(5.6)
Neonatal jaundice	4(7.8)	IUGR	2(3.7)
Respiratory distress	3(5.8)	Placenta previa	2(3.7)
Post-hemorrhagic hydrocephalus	1(2.0)	TTTS & IUFD	1(1.9)
Neonatal vomiting	1(2.0)	Invasive GAS infection & IUFD	1(1.9)
Total	51(100.0)	Ectopic pregnancy	1(1.9)
		Atonic bleeding	1(1.9)
		Traffic accident	1(1.9)
*: A pair of twins included		Total	54(100.0)

ELBW: extremely low birth weight <1000 g, PROM: premature rupture of the membranes, GAS: group A streptococcus, IUGR: intrauterine growth restriction, TTTS: twin-to-twin transfusion syndrome, IUFD: intrauterine fetal death.

Table 1. Reasons for neonatal and maternal transports (June 2003 – Dec 2010).

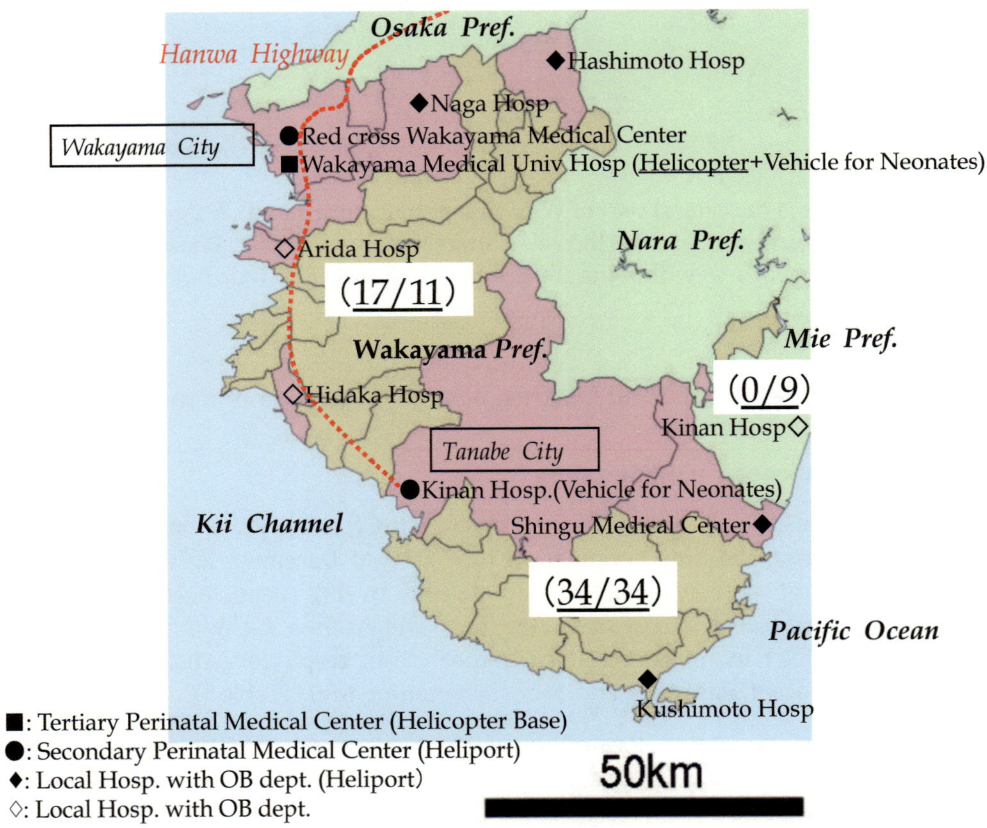

Fig. 2. Number of perinatal (neonatal/maternal) helicopter transports in Wakayama prefecture and southern Mie prefecture from June 2003 to December 2010, and the perinatal transport system in 2011.

3.2 Maternal helicopter transportation

There were 54 cases of maternal transfer (7.1 cases/year) by helicopter during the same time period. The reasons of transfer were threatened premature delivery (n=25), preterm premature rupture of membranes (PROM) (n=13), pregnancy-induced hypertension (PIH) (n=4), threatened abortion (n=3), intrauterine growth restriction (IUGR) (n=2), placenta previa (n=2), twin to twin transfusion snydrome (TTTS) & intrauterine fetal death (IUFD) (n=1), invasive group A streptococcus (GAS) infection & IUFD (n=1), ectopic pregnancy (n=1), atonic bleeding (n=1) and traffic accident (n=1) (Table 1). We transported one patient with threatened premature delivery and another with placenta previa from Shingu Medical Center in southeast Wakayama prefecture to Kinan hospital, a secondary perinatal medical center in south Wakayama with the helicopter. Two out of the 3 threatened or imminent abortions resulted in abortion. The patients with ectopic pregnancy and atonic bleeding, respectively, both survived. Six pregnant women with threatened premature delivery were back-transferred to their local hospitals overland once the condition stabilized. The other 42 patients, including four twin pregnancies, resulted in 45 live births (5.9 infants/year) in our hospital and one stillbirth due to maternal invasive GAS infection. Delivery after helicopter transfer was 42 (1.12 %) out of 3763 total deliveries in ten years. The referring facilities for all 54 patients were in north Wakayama (n=11), south Wakayama (n=34), and south Mie (n=9) (Fig. 2). The average time from receiving request of helicopter transport from a local hospital until take-off and return to site 13R was 19 ± 19 min and 1 hr, 20 ± 27 min, respectively.

An exception to the rule of inter-facility perinatal transport was made in the case of a patient at 36 weeks of pregnancy who was involved in a traffic accident. The patient had pneumothorax, femur fractures, and threatened premature delivery, and was transported from a primary school playground near the traffic accident site, based on a request by a paramedic. Caesarean section was performed soon after emergency medical treatment was completed.

3.3 Propagation of installing in-facility heliport

In-facility heliports have been installed in local hospitals since 2006 in Wakayama prefecture (Fig. 2). These are advantageous since there is no need for a local ambulance to transfer patients from a hospital to a heliport site outside the hospital. Thus, in-facility heliports simplify helicopter inter-facility transportation without using heliports outside the local hospital as a rendezvous point. Until February 2006, all neonatal (n=23) and maternal (n=19) helicopter transports occurred by way of non-hospital rendezvous points. After February 2006, in-facility heliports were used in 23 (82.1%) out of 28 cases of neonatal transports and 26 (74.3%) out of 35 cases of maternal transports (Fig. 1). Using the in-facility heliport, the time from landing at the site where patients were waiting to landing at the helicopter base on 13R of the hospital has been shortened 3 to 12 minutes compared to using the rendezvous points outside the hospital (Table 3).

4. Change in maternal and child health statistics after introduction of helicopter emergency medical service into perinatal transportation

There were 36 perinatal helicopter transports (16 maternal transports and 20 neonatal transports) in 2004-2006. The maternal transports comprised 9 from SW, 2 from NW and 5 from SM; and the neonatal transports comprised 13 from SW and 7 from NW (Table 4). Therefore, origin of perinatal helicopter transports in Wakayama Prefecture comprised of 29% from NW and 71% from SW, although SW had only 21% of the live births in Wakayama Prefecture in 2003. Live births-based frequency in perinatal helicopter was 9.3 times greater in SW than in NW. There were no accidents during transport and no requested flights were cancelled.

Time course in neonatal transport			
Heliport	*Outside the facility: n=28*	*In-facility: n=22*	
	Time from reception to lift-off		Difference
mean	0:19	0:26	0:07
median	0:11	0:22	0:11
	Time from reception to landing on the spot		Difference
mean	0:38	0:44	0:06
median	0:33	0:37	0:04
	Time from reception to landing on the base		Difference
mean	1:22	1:25	0:03
median	1:17	1:13	-0:04
Time course in maternal transport			
Heliport	*Outside the facility: n=24*	*In-facility: n=25*	
	Time from reception to lift-off		Difference
mean	0:12	0:19	0:07
median	0:10	0:17	0:07
	Time from reception to landing on the spot		Difference
mean	0:38	0:38	0:00
median	0:36	0:40	0:04
	Time from reception to landing on the base		Difference
mean	1:21	1:15	-0:06
median	1:20	1:12	-0:08

Table 3. Comparison of the transportation time course using in-facility heliport with the one using the rendezvous points outside the hospital.

Region	*South Wakayama*	*North Wakayama*	*South Mie*	*North Mie*
Area, km^2	2383.2(50.4%)	2342.92(49.6%)	991.74(17.2%)	4769.66(82.8%)
Population in 2003	207,200(19.6%)	850,263(80.4%)	88,075(4.7%)	1,776,110(95.3%)
Live births in 2003	1772(20.7%)	6789(79.3%)	566(3.4%)	15,931(96.6%)
Maternal transports	9	2	5	0
Neonatal transports	13	7	0	0

Table 4. Regional differences between southern and northern parts in Wakayama and Mie prefectures, and number of perinatal helicopter transports for 3 years from 2004 to 2006 in each region.

The gestation periods in the maternal air transports from SW and SM were 19 weeks in 1 case, 22-23 weeks in 4 cases, 24-27 weeks in 7 cases, and 28-31 weeks in 2 cases (Table 5). Twelve of the 14 maternal transports (86%) were performed at less than 28 weeks of gestation. The number of twin pregnancies was 2. Eight out of 14 (57%) of the babies were delivered in less than 7 days after transport. One case ended as stillbirth at 20 weeks' gestation. All four women who were air-transported at 22-23 weeks delivered in less than 7 days after air-transportation (Table 5).

Pregnancy	*No. of transport*	*No. of Delivery*	*Span between transport and delivery: Days*	*No. of mothers*
< 22W	1	1	< 1	3
22-23W	4*	4*	1~6	5*
24-27W	7*	4	7~13	0
28-31W	2	3*	14~30	4*
32-36W	0	0	31~60	1
37-41W	0	2	60 <	1
Total	14	14	Total	14

*: included 1 twin-pregnancy

Table 5. Gestation at transport and delivery, and span between transport and delivery in the maternal helicopter transports from South Wakayam and South Mie.

No anomalies were observed in the 15 infants born alive, but 9 of the 15 infants (60%) were extremely low-birth-weight (ELBW<1000 g) and one of these (11%) died. Three of the 13 neonatal air-transports (23%) from SW died due to ELBW + rupture of the liver capsule, severe asphyxia, and congenital heart disease, respectively (Table 6). There were no maternal deaths in the women transported by helicopter.

Outcome of maternal transports		
South Wakayama N= 9 (1: twin)	Stillbirth	0/1
	ELBW	5/5
	VLBW	3/3
	NBW	1/1
South Mie N=5 (1: twin)	ELBW	3/4
	LBW	1/1
	NBW	1/1
	Total	14/16

Outcome of neonatal transports		
South Wakayama N=13	CHD	4/5
	Birth asphyxia	2/3
	Neonatal jaundice	2/2
	ELBW	0/1
	Hydrocephalus	1/1
	Anal atresia	1/1
	Total	10/13

ELBW: extremely low birth weight, VLBW: very low birth weight, NBW: normal birth weight
CHD: congenital heart disease

Table 6. Outcome of infants after perinatal transportation. Number of infants discharged alive from NICU/number of infants admitted to NICU after perinatal helicopter transportation.

The neonatal and perinatal mortality rates for the three years (2004-2006) after introduction of helicopter transportation decreased by -0.31 and -0.57 in South Wakayama (SW), -0.28 and -0.18 in North Wakayama (NW), -0.90 and -2.49 in South Mie (SM), and -0.49 and -1.48

in North Mie (NM), respectively, compared to the three years before introduction of the helicopter (2000-2002) (Table 6). The differences in neonatal and perinatal mortality rates in 2004-2006 compared to 2000-2002 were greater in SW than in NW, and in SM compared to NM. The fetal death rate decreased by -0.78 in SW, -1.19 in NW, -1.59 in SM, and -2.65 in NM in 2004-2006 compared to 2000-2002, with greater decreases in NW than in SW, and in NM compared to SM. Fetal death rate in NW ($p<0.05$) and neonatal mortality rate ($p<0.01$), perinatal mortality rate ($p<0.01$), and fetal death rate ($p<0.01$) in NM all differed significantly between 2004-2006 and 2000-2002 (Table 7). The changes in the number of maternal deaths between 2000-2002 and 2004-2006 were 0 in SW, 1 in NW, -2 in SM, and -1 in NM, with the greatest change occurring in SM (Kumagai, et al., 2011)

Neonatal mortality	*2000-2002*	*2004-2006*	*Difference*	*95 %CI*
South Wakayama	2.14	1.84	-0.31	-0.362, 3.06
North Wakayama	1.44	1.16	-0.28	-0.98, 0.42
South Mie	1.5	0.597	-0.90	-3.04, 1.24
North Mie	1.78	1.29	-0.49*	-0.99, -0.01
Perinatal mortality	*2000-2002*	*2004-2006*	*Difference*	*95 %CI*
South Wakayama	4.45	3.88	-0.57	-3.05, 1.90
North Wakayama	5.10	4.92	-0.18	-1.54, 1.18
South Mie	5.46	2.97	-2.49	-6.74, 1.76
North Mie	6.03	4.55	-1.48**	-2.40, -0.56
Fetal death rate	*2000-2002*	*2004-2006*	*Difference*	*95 %CI*
South Wakayama	32.7	31.9	-0.78	-7.46, 5.89
North Wakayama	28.6	27.4	-1.19**	-4.34, 1.96
South Mie	30.0	28.4	-1.59	-12.36, 9.19
North Mie	28.0	25.3	-2.65**	-4.67, -0.64
No. of maternal deaths	*2000-2002*	*2004-2006*	*Difference*	
South Wakayama	1	1	0	
North Wakayama	0	1	1	
South Mie	2	0	-2	
North Mie	3	2	-1	

CI: confidence interval, *: $p<0.05$, **: $p<0.01$

Table 7. Differences in maternal and child health statistics between 3 years before (2000-2002) and after (2002-2004) introduction of perinatal helicopter transportation.

5. Discussion

Prefectural and national governments have a responsibility to maintain and improve perinatal medical care in Japan, and the efforts made at the prefectural level is reflected by the maternal and child health statistics. Maternal and child health care in Japan has reached a world-class level and is still improving year by year. In this study, a comparison of neonatal and perinatal mortalities between the three-year periods before and after introduction of helicopter transport for perinatal cases showed greater decreases in the southern parts of Wakayama and Mie Prefectures compared to the northern part of each prefecture. The southern parts of each prefecture are sparsely populated areas that are remote from each prefectural capital. The highest decrease in the number of maternal deaths occurred in South Mie, most likely due to the introduction of perinatal helicopter transport since all 5 helicopter transports from this region were maternal transports. Overall, the data suggest that perinatal transportation using a single "doctor-helicopter" in a sparsely populated area will contribute to improvement of maternal and child health despite the fact that statistical differences were not significant, as the areas involved are sparsely populated.

In a large metropolitan area in Southern California, a helicopter transport service has been used successfully to move emergency patients from referring hospitals to a perinatal center (Elliot JP, O'Keeffe DF & Freeman RK). Cooperation among helicopter transports overlapping each coverage area is important for improving perinatal medicine, especially for handling patients during a disaster. In 2010, Wakayama prefecture has secured flight cooperation for helicopter transports with neighboring Osaka and Tokushima prefectures (Fig. 2).

Maternal helicopter transport represented 1.12% of all deliveries in our hospital and the cause of it was threatened premature delivery, preterm premature rupture of membranes, and pregnancy-induced hypertension in numerical order. This order is the same as the report from Nova Scotia that the primary reasons for maternal air transfer representing 1.3% of all deliveries were threatened preterm labor (41%), preterm premature rupture of the membranes (21%), hypertensive disease/hemolysis, elevated liver enzymes, and low platelets (16.5%) in the Women's Hospital (Jony & Baskett, 2006).

One of the effects of maternal helicopter transport was a high rate of ELBW (58%) in infants born after transport from South Wakayama and South Mie, which does not necessarily mean that helicopter transport caused high rate of ELBW infants to the mothers transported. The gestation period in the cases of maternal transport was less than 28 weeks in 12 out of 14 women, and all 4 women at 22 or 23 weeks' gestation delivered within 7 days after transport. The pregnant women who were transported from distant local hospitals tended to have earlier pregnancy and earlier delivery after transport. The both factors seemed to lead to the high rate of ELBW.

Abortion is de facto legal in Japan, with some limitations. Approved doctors can virtually practice abortion to anyone after 12 and before 22 weeks gestation if consent was given by the mother. The decision to request maternal transport for high risk pregnancy tends to have been made in local hospitals after 22 weeks and 0 days of gestation, at which time abortion is redefined as preterm birth by the maternal health protection law amended in 1996.

A helicopter flight of 100 km is completed around 30 min and is less bumpy and invasive than ground transport for more than 3 hours (Ohara et al., 2008). However, hurried and noisy helicopter transport may add stress to pregnant women and lead to triggering of earlier delivery (American Academy of Pediatrics Section on Transport Medicine, 2007).

The fetal death rates in South Wakayama and South Mie remain higher than those in North Wakayama and North Mie. Since perinatal mortality rates are already lower in the southern areas compared to those in North Wakayama and North Mie, fetal deaths before 22 weeks gestation are thought to be a cause of the high rate in fetal death after 12 weeks of pregnancy). Fetal death is divided into spontaneous and artificial. The artificial fetal death rate in Japan has been higher than the spontaneous rate since 1984, and in 2006 these rates were 15.6 and 11.9, respectively. Socioeconomic problems in sparsely populated areas, such as fewer primary obstetric facilities, a higher maternal age (Salihu et al., 2008), and lower income (Nishi & Miyake, 2007) compared to urban areas, may be related to the higher fetal death rate.

6. Conclusion

Human resources in the fields of obstetrics and pediatrics have decreased in Japan, and patient transportation is important for maintaining the quality of perinatal medicine, especially in sparsely populated areas. The Helicopter Emergency Medical Service is of value in perinatal transportation and this approach is likely to be adopted nationally in Japan.

7. References

Department of Health and Welfare, Mie Prefecture. *Vital statistics in Mie,* Available from: <http://www.pref.mie.jp/DATABOX/>

Department of Health and Welfare, Wakayama Prefecture. *Vital Statistics in Wakayama,* Available from: <http://www.pref.wakayama.lg.jp/prefg/050100/dotai/>

Elliot JP, O'Keeffe DF & Freeman RK. (1982). Helicopter transportation of patients with obstetric emergencies in an urban area. *Am J Obstet Gynecol.* 143:157-62

Japanese Society for Aeromedical Services, (2011). Available from: < http://www.medianetjapan.com/2/town/government/airrescue/>

Jony L & Baskett TF. Emergency air transport of obstetric patients. (2007). *J Obstet Gynaecol Can.* 29:406-8.

Kumagai T, Higuchi R, Okutani T, et al., (2011). Change maternal and child health outcomes after introduction of a helicopter into perinatal transportation in Japan. *Mater Child Health J,* 15(2):255-9

Ministry of Health, Labor, and Welfare. *MHLW Statistical Database,* Available from: <http://wwwdbtk.mhlw.go.jp/toukei/>

Mothers' & Children's Health & Welfare Association, Eds. (2006). Notes, In: *Maternal and Child Health Statistics of Japan,* pp. (10-13). Mothers' & Children's Health Organization, ISBN978-4-89430-024-8, Tokyo Japan

Nishi M & Miyake H. (2007). Infant and perinatal mortalities and fetal deaths in household out of employment. *J Health Welfare Statistics (Jap).* 54: 34-38

Ohara M, Shimizu Y & Satou H, et al. (2008). Safety and usefulness of maternal transport using a helicopter. *J Obstet Gynecol Res.* 34: 189-194

Okutani T, Booka M, Kumagai K, et al. (2006). Perinatal helicopter transportation in Wakayama Prefecture. *Jap J Soc Perinat Neonat Med,* 42: 30-35

Salihu H, Wilson RE, Alio AP, et al. (2008). Advanced maternal age and risk of antepartum and intrapartum stillbirth. *J Obstet Gynecol Res.* 34: 843-850

Section on Transport Medicine American Academy of Pediatrics. (2007). Neonatal ICU Consideration. In: *Guidelines for air and ground transport of neonatal and pediatric patients* (3rd ed). Woodward DA, at al. (Eds), pp. (333-340), American Academy of Pediatrics, ISBN-10: 1-58110-219-4, IL U.S.A

Section on Transport Medicine American Academy of Pediatrics. (2007). Transport physiology and stresses of transport, In: *Guidelines for air and ground transport of neonatal and pediatric patients* (3rd ed), Woodward DA, at al. (Eds), pp. (197-218), American Academy of Pediatrics, ISBN-10: 1-58110-219-4, IL U.S.A

7

The Contribution of Severe Pre-Eclampsia and Eclampsia to Perinatal Mortality in a Nigerian Teaching Hospital

Olufemiwa Niyi Makinde
Dept. of Obstetrics, Gynaecology and Perinatology, College of Health Sciences, Obafemi Awolowo University, Ile-Ife, Nigeria

1. Introduction

The continuum of pre-eclampsia/eclampsia accounts for about one-third of maternal deaths in developing countries (Thomas, 1998).Perinatal deaths still occur preponderantly in low-income and middle-income countries and in places such as south Asia and sub-Saharan Africa, many of these occur during labor or birth. These are areas where, if the median proportion of births attended by skilled attendants were 100% rather than 49%, or if the median caesarean section was 24% instead of 3%, most of these tragedies would not have happened (Lawn, 2011).In each materno-fetal unit, the mother is like an "incubator" for the fetus. Perinatal outcome directly reflects the quality of existing obstetrical and neonatal services (Baveja, 2001, Lumley & Bakoula, 1993). Consequently, adverse outcomes to the mother during pregnancy and labour may impact negatively on the fetus and newborn resulting in perinatal death. A composite perinatal audit is the need of the hour for each obstetric unit so as to evolve a system of professional analysis of maternal and child health (MCH) services This study aims to: (i) highlight the magnitude of perinatal mortality among 39 consecutive cases of **severe pre-eclampsia/eclampsia(SPEE)**during the study period; (ii) classify perinatal deaths using the Tulip classification; (iii) to determine the effect of birthweight, antenatal care, multiple pregnancy and parity on perinatal death; (iv)to highlight the imperativeness of skilled attendance at birth on a 24 hour basis by using the workload indicator of staffing needs(WISN) concept; (v) to profer suggestions to accelerate progress for coverage of clinical-care interventions to stem the tide of intolerably high perinatal mortality rate among cases of **SPEE**.

2. Patients and methods

During the study period from 1st of January,2006 to 31st of January,2007, 39 consecutive cases of SPEE were admitted into the maternity unit of the Obafemi Awolowo University Teaching Hospitals Complex, Ile-Ife Nigeria. Each case on presentation was categorized into (1) severe pre-eclampsia, on the basis of hypertension after the 20th week of gestation, the diastolic blood pressure $\geq$110 mmHg on admission, proteinuria $\geq$30mg/dl in random urine specimen or $\geq$ 300mg in a 24hr urine specimen. (2) Imminent eclampsia, on account of parameters in (1) and symptoms of headache, blurring of vision and upper abdominal pain. (3) Eclampsia, existence of the parameters in (1) and occurrence of seizures.

The infant outcome of all the consecutive cases of **SPEE** admitted during the study period were determined. The perinatal mortality (**PNM**) rate associated with cases of SPEE was determined. Perinatal deaths were classified using the Tulip classification (6 main causes and 6 mechanisms). The 6 main causes of perinatal mortality were congenital anomaly, placental/umbilical disorders, prematurity, infection, others like fetal hydrops of unknown origin, maternal disease, trauma and unknown causes. Five expert observers (raters) namely 3 senior registrars in obstetrics,1 senior registrar in neonatology and 1 pathologist independently determined the most probable cause of perinatal death and the mechanism of such death for each case. Statistical analysis was by Stata version 11. Fleiss kappa was used to determine the degree of agreement beyond chance. Kappa value ranging from 0.81 - 1.00 indicates very good strength of agreement and value ranging from 0.21- 0.40 indicates fair agreement The 6 specified mechanisms for PNM are cardio-circulatory insufficiency, multi-organ failure, respiratory insufficiency, cerebral insufficiency, placental insufficiency and unknown causes. The effect of antenatal care, birth weight, multiple pregnancy and parity on perinatal mortality among the cohort of cases of SPEE was also determined.

The workload indicator for staffing need (WISN) ratio was also determined for the labour ward, labour ward theatre and neonatal intensive care unit. This is a WHO concept developed to show the adequacy or otherwise of available skilled attendants manning hospital units such as the labour/labour ward theatre delivery and neonatal care units. The patient load of the unit is determined and the job description for each cadre of skilled attendants is determined. From these, the required number of staff needed is calculated making provisions for sick leave, annual leave and off duty. The WISN ratio is calculated thus: ACTUAL number of staff on ground (numerator)/ REQUIRED (Calculated) number of staff(denominator). If the WISN ratio is < 1.0, the staff strength is inadequate. If the ratio is ≥ 1.0, the staff strength is adequate or more than enough.

3. Results

During the study period, there were 39 consecutive cases of SPEE with 43 infants delivered. The age of the mothers ranged from 18-38 years, 27(69.2%) were unbooked and the gestational age at presentation ranged from 22-41 weeks. The cases were severe pre-eclampsia 16 (41.02%), imminent eclampsia11(28.2%), eclampsia- antepartum 6(15.4%), intrapartum 2(5.1%), and postpartum 4(10.3%).10 (25.6%) of the mothers with SPEE had spontaneous vaginal delivery, 4(10.3%) had operative vaginal delivery while majority 25(64.1%) had lower segment Caesarean section.

Perinatal mortality among the women with severe preecalmapsia/eclampsia is shown in Table 1. There was 6 perinatal deaths among the four cases. Three early neonatal death were in a set of triplet. All the mothers with perinatal deaths were unbooked despite the fact that they were all high risk cases namely multiple pregnancy of higher fetal order, primigravidity, grand-multiparity and previous perinatal death. All the cases with perinatal death were also delivered preterm.

During the study period, there were 6 (13.95%) perinatal deaths out of 43 infants delivered by mothers with SPEE. The total births during the period were 1026. Consequently, the perinatal mortality rate associated with cases of SPEE (a single disease entity) during the study period was 5.84 per 1000 births.

S/N	AGE (Years)	Parity	E.G.A (Weeks)	Booking status	Diagnosis at presentation	Mode of Delivery	Infant outcome
1	31	P2	31	U	Eclampsia (Postpartum)	Spontaneous Vaginal Delivery	Triplets, Early neonatal death. All dead before arrival
2	21	P0	22	U	Eclampsia (Antepartum)	Spontaneous Vaginal Delivery	0.7kg; Male; Early neonatal death.
3	35	P5	31	U	Imminent Eclampsia	Spontaneous Vaginal Delivery	2.3kg; Male; Fresh Still Birth
4	30	P3	36	U	Imminent Eclampsia	Spontaneous Vaginal Delivery	2.8kg; Male; Fresh Still Birth

Table 1. Perinatal mortality among the women with severe preeclampsia/ eclampsia during the study period.

The causes of perinatal deaths among the cohort are in shown in Table 2a. It shows the level of agreement between the 5 expert raters concerning the cause of each perinatal death. While there was consensus that prematurity was the cause of perinatal death in the first 4 cases, the cause of perinatal death in cases 5 and 6 was agreed to be due to placenta and cord anomaly (Kappa = 1.00, z=7.75, p<0001). Showing a very good strength of agreement among the 5 expert observers as regards the most probable cause of death for each case.

Cases of Perinatal Mortality	Congenital Anomaly	Placenta and Cord Anomaly	Prematurity	Infection	Others	Unknown
Case 1	0	0	5	0	0	0
Case 2	0	0	5	0	0	0
Case 3	0	0	5	0	0	0
Case 4	0	0	5	0	0	0
Case 5	0	5	0	0	0	0
Case 6	0	5	0	0	0	0

Kappa = 1.00, z=7.75, p<0001

Table 2a.The causes of perinatal deaths among cases of SPEE by the experts according to Tulip classification.

Table 2b shows the mechanism for perinatal deaths according to the 5 expert raters.

Cases of perinatal Deaths	Cardio-pulmonary insufficiency	Multiple organ failure	Respiratory Insufficiency	Cerebral insufficiency	Placental insufficiency	Unknown
Case1	0	0	5	0	0	0
Case 2	0	0	5	0	0	0
Case 3	0	0	5	0	0	0
Case 4	0	0	4	1	0	0
Case 5	2	0	0	0	3	0
Case 6	2	0	2	0	1	0

Kappa= 0.36662, z=4.08,p=< 0.000.

Table 2b. Mechanisms of perinatal deaths among the women determined by the experts using Tulip classification.

All the 5 raters agreed that for cases 1,2 &3, the mechanism for perinatal death was respiratory insufficiency. For case 4,four raters agreed the mechanism was respiratory insufficiency while one thought it was due to cerebral insufficiency. For case 5, while two raters thought the mechanism was cardio-pulmonary insufficiency, remaining 3 thought it was due to placental insufficiency. For case 6, two raters each thought it was due to cardio-pulmonary and respiratory insufficiency respective while only one rater thought it was due to placental insufficiency (Kappa= 0.36662, z=4.08,p=< 0.000). Showing only a fair level agreement among the 5 expert observers.

The effect of antenatal care, birth weight, parity and multiple pregnancies on perinatal mortality among cases of SPEE is shown in table 3.

Factors assessed	Total no of infants	Perinatal death	Perinatal mortality (per 1000 total births)	P value
Antenatal Care				
Booked	8(18.6%)	0(0%)	0	
Unbooked	35(81.4%)	6(100%)	5.84	> 0.05
Birth weight				
<2.5kg	16(37.2%)	5(83.3%)	4.87	
≥2.5kg	27(62.8%)	1(16.7%)	0.97	< 0.05
Parity				
0	17(43.6%)	1(16.7%)	0.97	
1-4	21(53.8%)	4(66.8%)	3.89	
≥ 5	1(2.6%)	1(16.7%)	0.97	< 0.05
Multiple Pregnancy				
Singleton	36(83.7%)	3(50%)	2.92	
Twins	4(9.3%)	0	0	
Higher Order	3(7.0%)	3(50%)	2.92	<0.001

Table 3. Effect of antenatal care, birth weight, parity and multiple pregnancy on perinatal mortality among cases of SPEE.

Death was recorded only among those that were unbooked. However the difference between the two groups (booked vs unbooked was found not to be statistically significant. Low birth weight was also found to contribute significantly to perinatal death among the cohort. Though more number of perinatal deaths were recorded in nulliparae and grand-multiparae women compared to women of low parity, the difference was statistically not significant. Higher order pregnancies were also found to be to be a significant contributor to perinatal mortality.

Tables 4A, 4B and 4C shows the workload indicator for staffing need (WISN) in the labor ward, labor ward theatre and neonatal intensive care unit. The WISN ratio in the labour ward and labour ward theatre were 3.66 and 1.0 respectively. Average of three NIC unit personnel were available to take care of one neonate.

- Total no of births during the study period: 1026.
- Total no of days during the study period: 396.
- Delivery rate per day: 2.7(~3).
- Cadre and no of certified and experienced staff available per day:
  - Nurses/Midwives: 6(2per 8 hour shift).
  - Physicians: 5(*1 Consultant Obstetrician, 2 Senior Registrars,2 Registrars)
- Total no of heath care workers available **(actual)** within each 24 hour period: 11.
- **Require**d no of health care workers to attend to 2.7(~3) parturients within each 24-hour period=3.

Table 4A. The Workload Indicator for staffing need (WISN) in the labour ward.

- Total no of Caesarean sections(C/S) during the study period: 345.
- Total no of days during the study period: 396.
- Caesarean section rate per day: 345/396=0.87 (~1 C/S per day).
- Cadre and no of certified and experienced staff (minimum) that should handle a C/S:
  - Surgeons: 2
  - Perioperative Nurses: 2
  - Anaesthetists: 2.
  - Neonatologist: 1*(except when handling multiple pregnancies).
- Total minimum no of personnel required for a C/S in a teaching hospital: 7
- Total no of personnel available in the labour ward theatre within each 24 hour period for a C/S: 7.

Table 4B. The workload indicator for staffing need in the Labour ward theatre.

- Total no of neonates admitted during the study period: 311.
- Total no of days during the study period: 396.
- Neonatal admission rate per day: 311/396=0.78 (~1 neonate per day).
- Cadre and no of certified and experienced staff covering the NIC UNIT within each 24-hour period:
  - Physicians: 4(1 Consultant Neonatologist, 1 senior registrar,2 registrars.
  - Nurses: 8 (At least 2per 8hour shift).

Table 4C. The workload indicator for staffing need in the Neonatal Intensive Care Unit

4. Discussion

Maternal and fetal outcomes at birth are a sensitive indicator of the status of health systems so also are outcomes for newly born infants within the first week of extra-uterine life. Perinatal mortality is a severe adverse pregnancy outcome that involves death of the fetus in-utero (still-birth) as well as death of the newly born infant within the first week of life. The International Classification of Diseases, 10th revision (ICD-10) refers to fetal deaths and not stillbirths. Fetal death is defined as "death prior to the complete expulsion or extraction from its mother of a product of conception……. The fetus does not breathe or show any other evidence of life, such as beating of the heart, pulsation of the umbilical cord, or definite movement of voluntary muscles". The measurement focus is on fetal deaths in the last two trimesters of pregnancy and is defined by a birth-weight ≥ 500g;if birth-weight is unknown, by gestational age of ≥22 completed weeks; or, if both of these criteria are unknown, by crown-heel length of ≥ 25cm (WHO,ICD-10,1993).However, for international comparability, WHO recommends reporting of late fetal deaths (third trimester stillbirths at ≥1000g birth-weight,≥ 28 completed weeks of gestation, ≥35 cm body length)(WHO,1993).Nevertheless, it has also been recommended that outcomes at thresholds lower than 28 weeks may also be reported(WHO,2004). Globally, it has been estimated that about 2.6 million stillbirths occur annually (Cousens,2011).

The continuum of SPEE is still a highly recurrent obstetric complication in Ile-Ife, Nigeria and it has been noted to be accountable for about one-third of maternal deaths in developing countries (Thomas,1998;Makinde,2009). In the same hospital, an analysis revealed a perinatal mortality rate of 77.03 per 1,000 total births in 2003(Kuti,2003). This present study was therefore carried out to know the magnitude of the contribution of SPEE towards perinatal mortality within the hospital. The limitation of hospital based data in the correct assessment of the magnitude of a problem in a general population is recognized, the dearth of nationally collected vital statistics in most low-income countries has made regional surveys impracticable.

Table 1 shows the 6(13.9%) perinatal deaths out of 43 infants delivered by 39 females with SPEE. The perinatal mortality rate (PMR) attributable to SPEE was 5.8 per 1,000 total births since there were 1026 total births during the study period. From a single attributable factor, this PMR is intolerably high. It is noteworthy from Tables 1 and3, that all the 4 mothers with SPEE and 6 perinatal deaths never had ante-natal care (unbooked) whereas there was no perinatal death among the booked cases. All the 4 affected mothers with perinatal deaths were high risk cases namely multiple pregnancy of higher fetal order, primigravidity, grande-multiparity and previous history of perinatal death. Due to the lack of antenatal care by the affected mothers, there was no supervision of their pregnancies neither was there awareness about emergency preparedness and interventions which had dire consequences on their perinates.

Table2a shows the causes of the 6 perinatal deaths during the study period by the Tulip classification method. The first 4 cases were attributable to prematurity while the last 2 were due to placenta and cord anomalies. There was very good inter-rater agreement among the 5 observers with a Fleiss Kappa value of 1.00($z=7.77, p<0.0001$). The estimated gestational ages of the 6 cases of perinatal deaths ranged from 22-36 weeks. This is not surprising since the 4 affected mothers had life-threatening obstetric emergencies like eclampsia which would have necessitated delivery after initial stabilization. There were 2 fresh stillbirths which were adverse outcomes due to the maternal conditions.

Table2b shows the mechanism of the causes of death. The first 3(the triplets) were attributable to respiratory insufficiency while there were no perfect agreement for cases 4,5 and 6. Overall, the Fleiss Kappa value for mechanism for the causes of death was 0.36662 (z=4.08, p< 0.0001),this shows that there was fair inter-rater agreement. Knowing the causes of perinatal mortality is essential when designing interventions, and there are at least 35 published classification systems which makes comparison of the systems almost impossible or difficult. The Tulip classification for perinatal mortality allows unambiguous classification of underlying cause and mechanism, gives a good inter-rater agreement, with a low percentage of unknown causes and is easily applicable in a team of clinicians when guidelines are followed(Kortweq,2006).

The TULIP classification attempts to answer the question "why", while Wigglesworth system answers the question" when" and the RECODE answers the question "what". In order to answer these 3 questions related to perinatal mortality, there should be a combination of the classification systems (Kortweq, 2006; Gordjin,2009). Obviously, this would be cumbersome and may be unattainable in many health-care facilities especially in low-income countries.

Table 3A shows the glaring effect of antenatal care on perinatal mortality since antenatal care is one of the pillars of safe-motherhood. None of the booked cases recorded any perinatal death even though all the mothers had SPEE, however, the effect of antenatal care on perinatal mortality was not found to be statistically significant. Table3B shows that preponderantly, low birth-weight infants had a higher perinatal mortality rate(4.87compared with 0.97 per 1000 total births) and this was found to be statistically significant(p<0.05). Table 3C shows that parous mothers preponderantly experienced a perinatal mortality rate of 3.89 per 1,000 total births compared with 0.97 per 1000 total births respectively for both nulliparous and grande-multiparous mothers. There were more perinatal deaths associated with singleton and pregnancies of higher fetal order than in twins. This was found to be statistically significant with a p value<0.001.

The causes of maternal mortality are often inseparable from causes that lead to perinatal mortality (Pattinson et al, 2011). WHO has identified four main interventions which are critical in efforts to reduce maternal mortality in developing countries namely, family planning, antenatal care, skilled birth attendance and emergency obstetric care. Table 4A, B and C shows the workload indicator for staffing needs (WISN) in the labour ward, labour ward theatre and neonatal intensive care unit of the hospital.

Workload indicator for staffing need is a method that can help planners and managers estimate staff requirements, allocate staff among diverse health facilities, and monitor staff performance (Shipp,1998).The job description of each cadre of staff within a health-care facility to meet acceptable professional standards of service delivery is determined. Thus, the calculated (required) number of staff in a unit is determined based on their activities and compared with the number actually on ground using the WISN ratio. If the WISN ratio is 1.0, i.e actual staff equals calculated staffing requirement, then the current staff is just sufficient to meet the workload according to the professional standards which have been set. If the WISN ratio is < 1.0, then the current staff is not sufficient to meet the standards set and if the ratio is > 1.0, then there are more than enough staff to meet the standards set. Table 4 A, shows a WISN ratio of 3.66 for the labour ward of the hospital indicating that there are more than enough skilled attendants of different cadres to cope with the deliveries. Table 4B indicates that the labour-ward theatre had a WISN ratio of 1.0 indicating that the staffing strength was just enough to cope with basic and comprehensive emergency obstetric services in the unit.

Progression of pre-eclampsia to eclampsia is an obstetrical emergency. Hypertensive disease of pregnancy has been reported to have 20% antepartum and intrapartum stillbirth effects each(Bhutta,2011; Dolea,2003). It is therefore imperative to detect and manage hypertensive disease in pregnancy promptly and effectively as part of advanced antenatal care. However, this would be possible only if the affected pregnant females access care in a standard health-care facility thus community mobilization and education strategies for promotion of appropriate care seeking should be evolved. In low-income areas, poverty is prevalent, therefore, emergency loans through micro-insurance funds effected through public-private partnerships may be instituted for emergency obstetric care.

The availability of skilled birth attendants adequate numerically on a 24-hour basis is essential to stem the tide of intolerably high maternal and perinatal mortality and morbidity. For such skilled staff, there should be proficiency in partogram usage in labour and neonatal resuscitation and care. An earlier study in our community had shown that proficiency in partograph usage in labour can be achieved by lower cadre health care givers like community health extension workers especially in rural /semi-urban areas(Fatusin, et al,2008).

Prevention of a disease state and its complications is always better. In this study, 26/39 (66.6%) of the mothers were unbooked and a perinatal mortality rate of 5.84 per 1000 total births was recorded all in unbooked mothers. In many high income countries, the perinatal mortality is <10 per 1000 births from various causes. It is therefore glaring that from a single disease entity(SPEE), perinatal mortality rate of 5.84 per 1000 births is intolerably high. In an environment like this, the Pre-eclampsia Community Guidelines (PRECOG) recommendations when adhered to would go a long way in minimizing the incidence and complications of SPEE. The PRECOG provides an evidenced based risk assessment with criteria for early referral for specialist input, a two-tiered schedule for monitoring women in the community after 20 weeks of gestation and referral for stepped-up care(Milne,2005).Chemo-prophylaxis such as antenatal Calcium supplementation and low-dose aspirin(75mg) may also be beneficial in females at risk of hypertensive disease in pregnancy(Bhutta,2011; CLASP study,1994).

5. Conclusion

From this study, with a perinatal mortality rate of 5.84 per 1000 births attributable to a single disease entity, severe pre-eclampsia/eclampsia contributes significantly to perinatal mortality in our environment. Improvement of the quality and coverage of care to reduce maternal and perinatal deaths is complex as both are inextricably linked. Successful implementation of known lifesaving interventions within health system packages requires consideration of many interfaces between individual agents that affect whether the introduction of the packages will be effective. Every interface contributes to reduction of unnecessary deaths of mothers and their babies. There should also be a high degree of cooperation between policy makers, health promotion managers, the community, patients, health-care providers and managers within the health system to effect needed change to drastically reduce the high maternal and perinatal mortality in our environ.

6. References

Bhutta ZA, Yakoob MY, Lawn JE, Rizvi A, Friberg IK, Weissman E, Buckmann E, Goldenberg RI. tillbirths: what difference can we make and at what cost? The Lancet, April 2011; 65-80.

CLASP- A randomized trial of low dose aspirin for the prevention and treatment of pre-eclampsia among 9364 pregnant women, Farrel B for the collaboration Low dose Aspirin study in pregnancy collaborative Group. Lancet, 1994; 343:619-629.

Cousens S, Stanton C, Blencowe H, Stanton C, Chou D, Ahmed S, Steinhardt L,Creanga AA, Tuncalp O, Balsara ZP, Gupta S, Say L, Lawn JE. et al.ational, regional, and worldwide estimates of stillbirth rates in 2009 with trends since 1995: a systematic analysis. The Lancet 2011: Stillbirths: 13-24.

Fatusi AO, Makinde ON,Adeyemi AB, Orji EO, Onwudiegwu U. Evaluation of health workers' training in the use of the partogram. International Journal of Gynecology and Obstetrics,2008; 100: 41-44.

Gordjin SJ., Kortweq FJ., Erwich JT., Holn JP., van Diem MJ., Bergnon KA &Timnen A. Amultilayered approach for the analysis of perinatal mortality using different classification systems. Eur J Obstet Gynecol Reprod Biol,2009 Jun, 114(2): 99-104.

Kortweq FJ, Gordijn SJ, Timner A, Erwhich JJ, Berqman KA, Bouman K, Ravise JM, Herinqa MP and Holm JP.The Tulip classification of perinatal mortality; introduction and multidisciplinary inter-rater agreement. BJOG, 2006 Apr,113 (4):393-401.

Kuti O, Orji EO and Ogunlola IO.Analysis of perinatal mortality in a Nigerian teaching hospital. Journal of Obstetrics and Gynaecology, 2003; 23(5): 512-514.

Lawn JE., Blencowe H., Pattinson R., Cousens S., Kumar R., Ibiebele I., Gardosi J., Day LT & Stanton C,. Stillbirths: Where? When? Why? How to make the data count. The Lancet 2011; Stillbirths 2: 49-64.

Makinde ON, Adegoke OA, Adediran IA, Ndububa DA, Adeyemi AB, Owolabi AT, Kuti O, Orji EO and Salawu L. HELLP syndrome: the experience at Ile-Ife, Nigeria. Journal of Obstetrics and Gynaecology, 2009; 29(3): 195-199.

Milne F, Redman C, Walker J, Barker P, Bradley J, Cooper C, de Swiet M, Fletcher G, Jokinen M, Murphy D, Nelson-Piercy C, Osgood V. et al. The preeclampsia community guideline (PRECOG): how to screen for and detect onset of preeclampsia in the community. British Medical Journal, 2005; 330:576-580.

Pattinson R, Kerber K, Buchmann E, Friberg IK, Belizan M, Lansky S, Weissman E, Mathai M, Rudan I, Walker N, Lawn JE.et al. Stillbirths: how can health systems deliver for mothers and babies? The Lancet:April 2011; 81-94.

Shipp PJ (1998).Workload Indicator of staffing need. Prepared for the World Health Organization(1998),Dept. of Organization of Health Services Delivery(OSD), Geneva,Switzerland.

Thomas SV. Neurological aspects of eclampsia. Journal of the Neurological Sciences,1998: 155:37-43.

WHO. International statistical classification of diseases and related health problems: tenth revision, volume 2: instruction manual. Geneva: World Health Organization,1993.
WHO.ICD-10: International statistical classification of diseases and related health problems-instruction manual. Geneva, Switzerland: World Health Organization, 2004:2.

8

A Survey of Late Fetal Deaths in a Japanese Prefecture

Ryuzo Higuchi and Sawako Minami
Divisions of NICU and Obstetrics,
Department of Perinatal Medicine,
Wakayama Medical University
Japan

1. Introduction

Vital statistics in Japan show that the fetal death rate at ≥28 weeks gestation was 2.1/1000 live births in 2009 (Table 1), which is the lowest among high-income countries (Mother's & Children's Health & Welfare Association, 2011). Japan started to use 22 weeks instead of 28 weeks as a definition of late fetal death in 1995. Since these statistics started in 1947, the fetal death rate in Japan after 22 weeks gestation has been decreasing, and recently, the rate of decrease has slowed down since 2005. This is a common phenomenon among high-income countries, and especially in the UK, the late fetal death rate after 28 weeks gestation is actually starting to increase in the last few years. This is thought to be related to late child bearing and an increase in multiple births due to assisted reproductive technology in the UK (Confidential Enquiry into Stillbirths and Deaths in Infancy, 2001). Any 'child' expelled or issued forth from its mother after the 24th week of pregnancy that did not breathe or show any other signs of life is registered as a stillbirth in U.K., whereas a stillbirth after the 22nd week of pregnancy is registered as a late fetal death in Japan. Thus, there is a two-week difference in the definition of stillbirth between the U.K. and Japan, and medical interventions have been performed based on these definitions. The WHO general recommendation is 22 weeks of gestation.

Country	Year	Perinatal mortality rate	Fetal death rate at ≥28 weeks	Early neonatal mortality rate at < 7 days of age
Japan	2009	2.9	2.1	0.8
Singapore	2008	3.1	2.2	0.9
Sweden	2008	4.3	3.0	1.3
Italy	2007	4.5	2.8	1.7
Germany	2007	5.6	3.5	2.1
Netherlands	2007	5.8	3.4	2.4
U.S.A.	2003	6.8	3.1	3.7
U.K.	2003	8.5	5.7	2.8
France	2007	10.8	9.2	1.6

Table 1. Perinatal mortality rate in selected countries using fetal death rate at ≥28 weeks for international comparison.

Late fetal deaths at ≥22 weeks have outnumbered early neonatal deaths at < 7 days of age in the last 10 years (2000-2009) in the whole of Japan (77.9-80.7%) and in Wakayama prefecture (75.7-85.7%). Therefore, it is important to study risk factors or causes of late fetal deaths for prevention of these deaths and reduction of perinatal mortality. Obesity, socioeconomic status, and advanced maternal age in pregnancy have been listed as risk factors. Placental abruption, lethal congenital anomalies, infections, birth traumas, and blood type incompatibilities have been described as causes of late fetal death (Fretts, 2005). However, it is difficult to specify the cause of fetal death in a practical clinical setting, and the cause may be unknown in 25 to 60% of cases (Alessandri et al, 1992; Frøen et al, 2001; Huang et al, 2000; Yudkin et al, 1987). Even in a study with a 97% autopsy rate (Fretts, 1992), the causes of fetal death were unknown in 14% of the cases.

Using the new ReCoDe (relevant condition at death) classification, Gardosi et al. (2005) found that intrauterine growth restriction (FGR) was the cause of fetal death in 57.7% of cases classified as due to unknown causes using the conventional classification by Wigglesworth et al. (1980). The ReCoDe classification is based on the relevant condition at death. It does not mean the basic cause of fetal death. We surveyed late fetal deaths by means of a questionnaire mailed to obstetricians or midwives in all labor institutes in Wakayama prefecture, one of the 47 administrative divisions of Japan, which has a population of 1.000 million and live births of 7,516 in 2009. Data were examined using the ReCoDe classification, with the goal of obtaining results that will be useful for reducing the perinatal mortality rate in Japan and compensating for the dwindling birthrate in Japan.

2. Methods

We surveyed late fetal deaths, which were defined as stillbirths after 22 weeks of gestation, every year from 2001 to 2010 in Wakayama prefecture using a questionnaire mailed to obstetricians or midwives in all labor institutes in the prefecture. We mailed the questionnaire in March or April every year and requested a report on late fetal deaths in the previous year, including data and conditions that the obstetrician or midwife in charge considered to be most relevant to stillbirth. The requested data included the date of delivery, gestational age, the baby's birth weight and sex, maternal characteristics, and pregnancy details. The questionnaire collection was completed by the end of June. The cases were classified according to the ReCoDe classification using the data of the questionnaire obtained from the obstetrician or midwife in charge of them who reviewed the case record. The ReCoDe classification system seeks to establish what went wrong, but not necessarily why. The hierarchy of classification starts from conditions affecting the fetus and moves outwards in simple anatomical groups to those affecting umbilical cord, placenta, amniotic fluid, uterus, mother, intrapartum, trauma, and unclassified, which are subdivided into pathophysiological conditions, with the primary condition being the first on the list that is applicable to a given case. More than one category can be coded if the information is available. Intrauterine growth restriction is included as the last category in group A (A7): a fetus below the 10th percentile is assigned this classification only if no other specific fetal conditions are present (Committee of Neonate, Japan Pediatric Society, 2010). All cases were divided into groups of primipara and multipara pregnancies and the relationships between the parity and the relevant conditions for fetal death were compared by Fisher's direct method.

3. Results

Sixteen to 35 late fetal deaths (stillbirths after 22 weeks of gestation) per year from 2001 to 2010 were reported from 27-30 facilities in Wakayama prefecture. The total was 240 cases in the 10-year period. The mean response rate for the questionnaires mailed yearly to obstetricians and midwives in all labor institutes in the prefecture was 0.843 (0.743-0.933). There were 81425 live births and 303 late fetal deaths in Wakayama prefecture during the 10 years from 2001 to 2010, according to the vital statistics based on residence (Vital statistics in Japan, Tokyo: Ministry of Health, Labor and Welfare, 2010).

In the ReCoDe classification, the most frequent condition associated with late fetal death was intrauterine growth restriction (FGR) (A7) (n=73, 30.4%); followed by umbilical cord abnormalities excluding prolapse, entanglement, knot, and velamentous insertion (n=29, 12.1%); unexplained antepartum stillbirths (n=27, 11.2%); lethal congenital anomaly (n=27, 11.2%); placental abruption (n=26, 10.8%); intrapartum asphyxia (n=15, 6.3%); and twin-twin transfusion (n=15, 6.3%) (Table 2).

Primary ReCoDe classification		Year	01-05	06-10	01-10	%
A,	1. Lethal congenital anomaly	A1	16	11	27	11.3
Fetus	2. Infection, 2.1 Chronic	A2.1			0	0
	2.2 Acute	A2.2	1	1	2	0.8
	3. Non-immune hydrops	A3		2	2	0.8
	4. Isoimmunisation	A4			0	0
	5. Fetomaternal transfusion	A5			0	0
	6. Twin-twin transfusion	A6	7	8	15	6.3
	7. Fetal growth restriction	A7	35	38	73	30.4
B,	1. Prolapse	B1	2	2	4	1.7
Umbilical	2, Constricting loop or knot	B2	2	2	4	1.7
cord	3. Veramentous insertion	B3	1		1	0.4
	4. Umbilical cord-other	B4	13	16	29	12.1
C,	1. Abruptio	C1	11	15	26	10.8
Placenta	2. Previa	C2	1		1	0.4
	3. Vasa previa	C3	1		1	0.4
	4. Placental insufficiency	C4			0	0
	5. Placenta-other	C5		1	1	0.4
D,	1. Chorioamnionitis	D1		1	1	0.4
Amniotic	2. Oligohydramnios	D2		1	1	0.4
fluid	3. Polyhydramnios	D3		1	1	0.4
E,	1. Rupture	E1	3		3	1.3
Uterus	2. Uterine anomalies	E2			0	0
	3. Uterus-other	E3		1	1	0.4

Primary ReCoDe classification		Year	01-05	06-10	01-10	%
F,	1. Diabetes	F1	1		1	0.4
Mother	2. Thyroid diseases	F2			0	0
	3. Essential hypertension	F3			0	0
	4. Hypertensive diseases in pregnancy	F4	2		2	0.8
	5. Lupus or antiphospholipid syndrome	F5			0	0
	6. Chorestasis	F6			0	0
	7. Drug misuse	F7			0	0
	8. Other maternal condition	F8		2	2	0.8
G,	1. Asphyxia	G1	9	6	15	6.3
Intrapartum	2. Birth trauma	G2			0	0
H,	1. External	H1			0	0
Trauma	2. Iatrogenic	H2			0	0
I,	1. No relevant condition identified	I1	13	14	27	11.3
Unclassified	2. No information available	I2			0	0
	Total		118	122	240	100.0

Table 2. Primary ReCoDe classification for 240 late fetal deaths in 2001-2010 in Wakayama prefecture.

There was no major change in the number of each primary ReCoDe classification between the first 5 years (total 118) and the latter 5 years (total 122) during the 10 years form 2001 to 2010.

A second ReCoDe class was found in 86 cases (35.8%). Among 73 cases whose primary ReCoDe classification was FGR (since FGR was the first on the list), 48 (65.8%) had a second category, with umbilical cord-other (B4) (n=21) and placental abruption (C1) (n=10) being the most frequent second ReCoDe category for FGR (A7) (Table 3). FGR was the second ReCoDe category in 19 (70.4%) of the 27 cases of lethal congenital anomalies (A1), 1 of 2 acute infections (A2.2), 1 of 2 non-immune hydrops (A3), and 6 (40%) of 15 twin-twin transfusions.

(A7) FGR	n=73
(A7) alone	n=25
(A7) with 2nd ReCoDe	n=48
(B2) Constricting loop or knot	3
(B3) Veramentous insertion	1
(B4) Umbilical cord-other	21
(C1) Placental abruption	10
(C2) Placenta previa	3
(C4) Placental insufficiency	1
(D3) Polyhydramnios	2
(E3) Uterus-other	1
(F4) Hypertensive diseases	2
(F8) Other maternal condition	1
(G1) Intrapartum aspyhxia	3

Table 3. Second ReCoDe categories in cases with FGR as the primary ReCoDe class.

The time of stillbirth was divided into 7 groups at three weeks intervals. The number of late fetal deaths was highest in weeks 22-24 of gestation, decreased gradually in weeks 25 to 30, and increased again in weeks 34 to 39. Late fetal death due to placental abruption occurred most often from 34 to 36 weeks of gestation (Fig. 1).

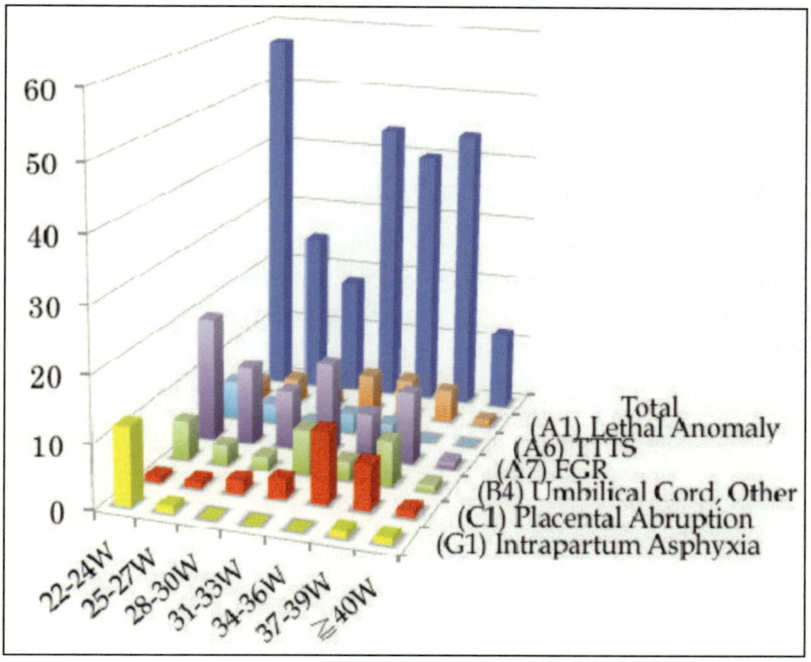

Fig. 1. Frequency of major ReCoDe categories according to gestational age.

A comparison of the causes of late fetal death in multipara and primipara cases showed that placental abruption was a more frequent cause in multipara cases (OR 3.64 [95%CI 1.47-9.02]), whereas FGR was a less frequent cause in multipara cases (OR 0.43 [95%CI 0.24-0.77]) (Table 4). Hypercoiled cord was most frequent in the umbilical cord-other category in the ReCoDe classification (15/29) (Table 5).

	Primipara n=129	Multipara n=111	Odds ratio	95% Confidence limit
(A1) Anomaly	18	9	0.54	[0.23-1.27]
(A6) TTTS	8	7	1.02	[0.36-2.90]
(A7) FGR	49	24	0.45	[0.25-0.80]
(B4) Umbilical cord-other	15	14	1.10	[0.50-2.39]
(C1) Abruptio	7	19	3.60	[1.45-8.92]
(G1) Asphyxia	5	10	2.46	[0.81-7.41]

Table 4. Odds ratio for major ReCoDe categories in multipara cases compared to primipara cases.

(B4) Umbilical cord-other	n=29
Hypercoiled	13
Stricture	5(1)
Torsion	2(1)[1]
Single Umbilical Artery	2
Umbilical Vein Thrombosis	1
Umbilical Cord Ulcer	1
Short Umbilical Cord	1
Unspecified	4

( ): number of cases combined with hypercoiled cord
[ ]: number of cases combined with single umbilical artery

Table 5. Items in the umbilical cord-other category.

Intrapartum asphyxia in babies from 22 to 23 weeks of gestation was the highest in the intrapartum asphyxia group (12/15) (Table 6). Unspecified multiple anomalies were most frequent and 18 trisomy was the second most common condition in the congenital lethal anomaly category (Table 7).

(G1) Intrapartum asphyxia	n=15
vaginal delivery at 22, 23 weeks gestation	12
vaginal delivery at 25 weeks gestation	1
Shoulder dystocia	1
Transverse lie	1

Table 6. Items in the intrapartum asphyxia category.

(A1) Lethal congenital anomaly	n=27
Unspedified multiple anomalies	10
18 trisomy	7
13 trisomy	3
Cardiac anomalies	3
Anencephaly	2
Other	2

Table 7. Items in the lethal congenital anomaly category.

There were 51 cases (21.3%) of advanced maternal age in pregnancy (≥35 years old) and the causes of late fetal deaths were FGR (n=12, 23.5%), placental abruption (n=9, 17.6%), umbilical cord-other (n=7, 13.7%), lethal anomaly (n=4, 7.8%) and unclassified (n=9, 17.6%).

There were 20 cases (8.5%) of pregnancies with assisted reproductive technology (ART). The mean maternal age in these cases was 35.0 years old, compared to 29.9 years old for non-ART pregnancies. ART included IVF-ET (n=12), AIH + ovulation inducer (n=4), AIH (n=2) and unspecified (n=2). The causes of late fetal deaths were FGR (n=9, 45%), lethal anomaly (n=3, 15%), uterus rupture (n=2, 10%), velamentous insertion (n=1, 5%), placental abruption (n=1, 5%), umbilical cord-other (n=1, 5%), and unclassified (n=3, 15%). Two of the 3 cases of uterus rupture (E1) involved pregnancies with ART, including one with AIH and one with an unspecified technique.

4. Discussion

A retrospective review of records is often a weak design due to lack of information recorded. In order to reduce this risk, this study was based on the yearly surveys obtained from the doctors or midwives in charge of the late fetal deaths who reviewed the previous year's records. The mothers were residents in Wakayama prefecture in 220 of the 240 cases of late fetal deaths reported in our survey. The custom of home-return for delivery, in which pregnant women give delivery in their home town where their parents can support them and care for their baby, is still partially alive in Japan, and this is the main reason why data from delivery institutes in a certain area do not coincide with the vital statistics in that area. However, the results of our survey are presumed to reflect the actual conditions of fetal deaths in Wakayama prefecture because we identified 220 (72.6%) of the 303 fetal deaths reported in the vital statistics.

We classified late fetal deaths according to the newly developed ReCoDe system (Gordosi et al, 2005) and found that the most frequent cause of late fetal death was FGR. This result is similar to that in a population-based cohort study performed in 1997-2003 in the West Midlands, U.K. (Gordosi et al, 2005).

The second most frequent cause of late fetal death in our survey was clearly an umbilical cord abnormality, excluding prolapse, constricting loop or knot, and velamentous insertion (B4), and these cases mainly involved a hypercoiled cord. There was no definition of hypercoiled cord in the questionnaire used in the survey. The obstetrician or midwife in charge reported conditions that they considered the most relevant to stillbirth and B4 ranked as the second most frequent cause of late fetal death. This is consistent with a report in Japan that 45% late fetal deaths are related to umbilical cord abnormality and that more than half of these cases involved a hypercoiled cord (Hasegawa et al, 2008). A hypercoiled cord has also been related to fetal death, fetal distress, meconium staining, and FGR in other studies (de Laat et al, 2007; Kashanian et al, 2005; Strong et al, 1994). Umbilical cord-other (n = 21) and placental abruption (n = 10) were the most common of the 48 second ReCoDes for FGR. To assess umbilical coiling, the umbilical coiling index (UCI) can be measured by ultrasound (Degani et al, 1995), but the sensitivity of the UCI for detection of hypercoiled cord at birth is only 17.3-25.4% (Quin et al, 2002; Predanic et al, 2005) and this method requires further development before it can be reliably used clinically to assess hypercoiled cord in utero.

Placental abruption is a serious emergency for both mother and child and is also highly unpredictable (Gordosi et al, 2005). The incidence of labor with placental abruption is highest at around 39 weeks of pregnancy, which is slightly earlier than for pregnancies without this complication (Ananth et al, 2001). The incidence of stillbirth with placental abruption peaked at 34-35 weeks of gestation in our survey, 4-5 weeks earlier than 39 weeks of gestation. We could not find any information that explained this difference in this survey. Overall, these results suggest that placental abruption may develop frequently from 34 to 39 weeks gestation, but perhaps in different ways in cases of late fetal death and live birth. In addition, multipara cases were more frequently associated with late fetal death due to placental abruption, compared to primipara cases. This does not necessarily mean that multipara pregnancies have a higher risk for placental abruption, since this study was based only on cases of late fetal death. Cohort studies and case controlled studies (Ananth et al, 1996. Kramer et al, 1997.

Sanchez et al, 2006) have been conducted in this regard, but these have produced different results for the risk of placental abruption with higher parity, with some showing no difference in the incidence of placental abruption between primipara and multipara pregnancies. Therefore, further studies are needed to reach a conclusion on this issue.

Twelve of 15 intrapartum asphyxias occurred in weeks 22-23 of gestation. Mortality in infants born at 22-23 weeks gestation has recently decreased in Japan, but the rate of major handicaps such as neurodevelopmental delay, cerebral palsy, visual impairment and hearing impairment are yet to improve (Hintz et al, 2005. Lorentz et al, 1998).

There are different policies on how to resuscitate babies born at 22-23 weeks gestation among delivery facilities in Japan. Babies with at least 24 weeks gestation are resuscitated at perinatal centers. If resuscitation at 22-23 weeks gestation becomes widely accepted in the near future in Japan, these fetal deaths will disappear or change to neonatal death. Intrapartum asphyxia at 22-23 weeks gestation may also affect the rate of late fetal death. Therefore, evaluation of the yearly change in late fetal death requires careful observation of the number of babies at 22-23 weeks gestation included in the sample population. We were unable to evaluate the extent of the risk of each abnormal condition because our survey was not performed as a cohort study that included all pregnancies in Wakayama or as a case controlled study with live births. However, this study does provide useful information for understanding the causes of late fetal deaths and for developing approaches for future prevention of these deaths.

5. Conclusion

Our data suggest that clinical follow up is important for placental abruption in multiparous pregnancy during weeks 34 and 36, for cord abnormalities (especially a hypercoiled cord) after 22 weeks gestation, and for primiparous pregnancy with FGR in order to decrease the late fetal deaths.

6. Summary

We surveyed late fetal deaths, defined as stillbirths after 22 weeks of gestation, from 2001 to 2010 in Wakayama prefecture using a questionnaire mailed to obstetricians and midwives in all labor institutes in the prefecture, one of the 47 administrative divisions of Japan. In the ten-year period, 240 stillbirths occurred and they were categorized using the ReCoDe (relevant condition at death) classification. The most common condition was intrauterine growth restriction (FGR) (n=73, 30.4%); followed by umbilical cord abnormalities such as a hypercoiled cord, excluding prolapse, entanglement, knot, and velamentous insertion (n=29, 12.1%); unexplained antepartum stillbirths (n=27, 11.3%); lethal congenital anomaly (n=27, 11.3 %); placental abruption (n=26, 10.9%); intrapartum asphyxia (n=15, 6.3%); and twin-twin transfusion (n=15, 6.3 %). A hypercoiled cord (n=15/29, 51.7%) was the most frequent condition in the umbilical cord category. Twelve of 15 stillbirths with intrapartum asphyxia occurred from 22 to 23 weeks gestation. The number of stillbirths with placental abruption peaked in the period from 34 to 36 gestational weeks (n=11/26, 42.3%). Multiparous women had a higher rate of placental abruption as the relevant condition at fetal death compared to primiparous women (OR 3.60 [1.45-8.92]), whereas fetal growth restriction was less common in multiparous women (OR 0.45 [0.25-0.80]).

7. References

Alessandri LM, Stanley FJ, Newnham J, et al. (1992). The epidemiological characteristics of unexplained antepartum stillbirths. *Early Hum Dev,* 30(2) : 147-61

Ananth CV, Wilcox AJ, Savitz DA, et al. (1996). Effect of maternal age and parity on the risk of uteroplacental bleeding disorders in pregnancy. *Obstet Gynecol,* 88(4 Pt 1): 511-6

Ananth CV, Wilcox AJ. (2001). Placental abruption and perinatal mortality in the United States. *Am J Epidemiol,* 153(4): 332-7

Committee of neonate, Japan Pediatric society. (2010). The new referential range of body constitution at birth by gestational age. *J Jap Pediatr Soci,* 114:1771-1806

Confidential enquiry into stillbirths and deaths in infancy: 8th annual report. (2001). CESDI; 2001, London

Degani S, Lewinsky RM, Berger H, et al. (1995). Sonographic estimation of umbilical coiling index and correlation with Doppler flow characteristics. *Obstet Gynecol,* 86(6) : 990-3

de Laat MW, van der Meij JJ, Visser GH, et al. (2007). Hypercoiling of the umbilical cord and placental maturation defect: associated pathology? *Pediatr Dev Pathol,* 10(4): 293-9

Fretts RC, Boyd ME, Usher RH, et al. (1992). The changing pattern of fetal death, 1961-1988. *Obstet Gynecol,* 79(1): 35-9

Fretts RC. (2005). Etiology and prevention of stillbirth. *Am J Obstet Gynecol,* 193(6): 1923-35

Frøen JF, Arnestad M, Frey K, et al. (2001). Risk factors for sudden intrauterine unexplained death: epidemiologic characteristics of singleton cases in Oslo, Norway, 1986-1995. *Am J Obstet Gynecol,* 184(4): 694-702

Gardosi J, Kady SM, McGeown P, et al. (2005). Classification of stillbirth by relevant condition at death (ReCoDe): population based cohort study. *BMJ* 331(7525): 1113-7

Gordijn SJ, Korteweg FJ, Erwich JJ, et al. (2009) A multilayered approach for the analysis of perinatal mortality using different classification systems. *Eur J Obstet Gynecol Reprod Biol,* 144(2): 99-104

Hasegawa J. (2008). Studies for early identification of umbilical cord abnormalities and for managements of high risk pregnancies with them. *Acta Obstet Gynaecol Jpn,* 60: 1723-34

Hintz SR, Kendrick DE, Vohr BR, et al. (2005). National Institute of Child Health and Human Development Neonatal Research Network. Changes in neurodevelopmental outcomes at 18 to 22 months' corrected age among infants of less than 25 weeks' gestational age born in 1993-1999. *Pediatrics,* 115(6): 1645-51

Huang DY, Usher RH, Kramer MS, et al. (2000). Determinants of unexplained antepartum fetal deaths. *Obstet Gynecol,* 95(2): 215-21

Kashanian M, Akbarian A, Kouhpayehzadeh J. (2006). The umbilical coiling index and adverse perinatal outcome. *Int J Gynaecol Obstet,* 95(1): 8-13

Kramer MS, Usher RH, Pollack R, et al. (1997). Etiologic determinants of abruptio placentae. *Obstet Gynecol,* 89(2): 221-6

Lorenz JM, Wooliever DE, Jetton JR, et al. (1998). A quantitative review of mortality and developmental disability in extremely premature newborns. *Arch Pediatr Adolesc Med,* 152(5): 425-35

Mother's & Children's Health & Welfare Association. (2011). *Vital statistics in Japan, 2010.* Mother's & Chidren's Health Organization, ISBN987-4-89430-024-8, Tokyo. Available from: http://www-bm.mhlw.go.jp/index.html

Predanic M, Perni SC, Chasen ST, et al. (2005). Assessment of umbilical cord coiling during the routine fetal sonographic anatomic survey in the second trimester. *J Ultrasound Med,* 24(2): 185-91

Qin Y, Lau TK, Rogers MS. (2002). Second-trimester ultrasonographic assessment of the umbilical coiling index. *Ultrasound Obstet Gynecol,* 20(5): 458-63

Sanchez SE, Pacora PN, Farfan JH, et al. (2006). Risk factors of abruptio placentae among Peruvian women. *Am J Obstet Gynecol,* 194(1): 225-30

Strong TH Jr, Jarles DL, Vega JS, et al. (1994). The umbilical coiling index. *Am J Obstet Gynecol,* 170(1 Pt 1): 29-32

Yudkin PL, Wood L, Redman CW. Risk of unexplained stillbirth at different gestational ages. Lancet 1987; 1(8543): 1192-4

9

Super Eyes and Hands for Future Fetal Intervention

Hiromasa Yamashita, Takashi Kakimoto, Wenji Yuan and Toshio Chiba
National Center for Child Health and Development
Japan

1. Introduction

With development of prenatal imaging technology diagnosis of fetal and placental disorders are becoming widely accepted in the field of perinatology especially so when some fetal condition may deteriorates before delivery. Awareness of prenatal conditions that may deteriorate before delivery or worsens soon after delivery is invaluable in planning long-term postnatal medical care. The idea of treating a fetus as a patient should never be considered strange or unusual any longer. If the affected fetuses do not undergo any treatment prenatally, devastating complications and/or deaths are likely to ensue.

Fetal surgical procedures are categorized into three categories of ; open surgery (with hysterotomy), endoscopic surgery (without hysterotomy), and ultrasound surgery. Using these procedures, prevention of fetal or neonatal mortality has been increasingly achieved promoting the chances of successful postnatal treatment with improved long-term quality of life. Endoscopic surgery is expected to correct fetal abnormalities using relatively simple modalities. An example of a simple and effective endoscopic surgery is the use of fetal tracheal occlusion to prevent intrauterine progression of pulmonary hypoplasia in congenital diaphragmatic hernia (CDH). As fetuses do not breathe *in utero*, this treatment's usefulness and importance cannot be overstated. Unlike this procedure, ex utero intrapartum treatment (EXIT), fetal myelomeningocele (MMC) repair, fetal lobectomy for congenital cystic adenomatoid malformation (CCAM), and fetal resection of sacrococcygeal teratoma (SCT) have been based on open procedure. The goal of these procedures is a long-term improvement of postnatal quality of life in case of MMC, and to save the fetal life in case of CCAM or SCT.

Fetal surgery is typically performed on fetuses around 19 to 28 weeks of gestation. The purpose is to treat fetal and placental morphologic defects, which could be diagnosed early before birth, and inhibit their progressions to point of sever fetal compromise. However, it may be complicated by surgical infections, premature labor, premature birth and membrane ruptureThe recent introduction of endoscopic and ultrasound image-guided surgeries have enabled minimally invasive intrauterine surgery (Harrison et al., 2001) thus reducing these potential complications of open fetal surgery to the barest minimum.

Our major target diseases are fetal CDH, fetal MMC, twin-to-twin transfusion syndrome (TTTS) and hypoplastic left heart syndrome (HLHS) or HLHS with restrictive atrial septum that inevitablly leads to irreversible pulmonary vascular damages. MMC is a dorsal neural tube defect with highest risk of hydrocephalus as well as motor/perception and vesico-rectal disabilities. Although current fetal repair of MMC is to surgically cover and protect the lesion *in utero*, this procedure is hard to accomplish endoscopically with the use of conventional surgical devices alone (Bruner et al., 1999; Kohl et al., 2006), as a result of a cramped working. TTTS occurs in 10-15% of monochorionic twin gestations and is caused by placental vascular anastomoses, resulting in an imbalance in blood flow and volume between both twins. In severely affected cases, this syndrome is likely to be associated with high perinatal mortality or postnatal life-long handicaps (Feldstein et al., 2000). As a definitive prenatal treatment, fetoscopic laser photocoagulation of the anastomotic vessels has been widely accepted (Senat et al., 2004; Quintero et al., 2000). Current procedures for correction of restrictive fetal atrial septum are still invasive because they require ultrasound-guided puncture of tiny beating fetal heart (Kohl et al., 2000; Marshall et al., 2004; Mäkikallio et al., 2006).

In order to overcome the challenges of fetal endosciopic surgery, improve surgical outcome and allow for more advanced surgery , we developed sets of new devices that will act as super eyes, super hand and improve navigation. We called them "super eyes", "super hands" and "super navigations".

In this chapter, we present details of these super devices and their applications for future fetal intervention. These technologies is sure to be employed both for stand-alone and combined use.

2. Super eyes

An ideal super eyes for intrauterine surgery should be able to exapand the views of the conventional endoscopic and ultrasound machine for preoperative diagnosis, intraoperative activities and visualisation of the operative field as well as postoperative monitoring Achieving this requires the use of high performance endoscopes and high-resolution 3D/4D ultrasound machine . We developed new endoscopes and ultrasound machines that perform the function of super eyes.

2.1 Three-dimensional fetoscope

Inside the uterus, fetal bodies and placental tissues are fragile and delicate. The Surgeon must be careful about manipulating surgical instruments, however conventional fetoscopes give only a two-dimensional (2D) view without depth perception. To solve this issue, we developed a miniature three-dimensional (3D) fetoscope of 5.4-mm diameter mounting double 1/10-inch CCDs and lens-units on the distal-end tip including a laser fiber channel of 1-mm diameter for safe laser photocoaguration (Fig. 1) (Kobayashi et al., 2009). This fetoscope can supply surgeons with a 3D front or a diagonally front view without any eye fatigue, enabling safe procedures in the uterus.

2.2 Fluorescence endoscope

In TTTS therapy, surgeons must assess anastomotic communicating blood vessels. However, small vessels are often missed due to the poor view which obtained with a fetoscope.

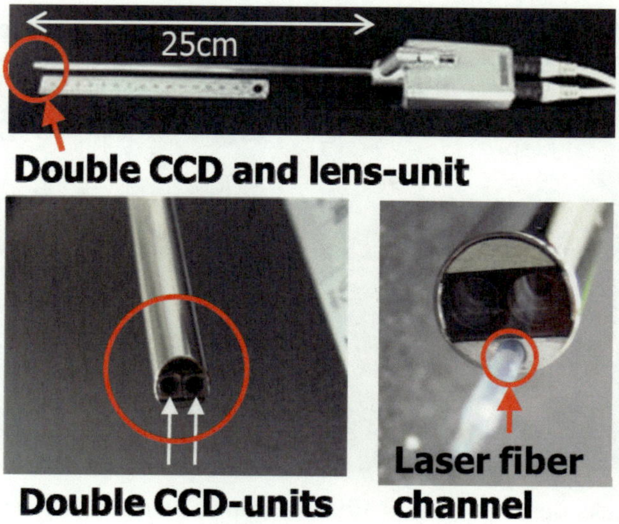

Fig. 1. Appearance of the 3D fetoscope. Miniature double CCD and lens-unit are in the distal-end tip to receive right-eye view and left-eye view. We developed another type of 3D fetoscope with a laser fiber channel.

To help this assessment, we developed a fluorescence endoscope which is capable of visualizing very small vessels, even in the cloudy amniotic fluid (Harada et al., 2009; Ishiyama et al., 2011). We did *in vitro* test to visualize a placenta of cynomolgus monkey. After the injection of indocyanine green (ICG) into the vessel, the endoscope can detect near-infrarede fluorescence (peak: 845 nm) from the vessels on the placenta in fluorescence mode of the camera. (Fig. 2).

2.3 Ultra-high sensitive endoscope

A conventional endoscope needs high-powered light to see inside the uterus. Using this light raises concern about causing negative effect to perinatal fetal ocular development by the intense heat and illumination. Therefore, we developed an ultra-high sensitive endoscope using High-gain Avalanche Rushing amorphous Photoconductor (HARP) camera technology, which has been originally developed by Japan Broadcasting Corporation (Nippon Hoso Kyoukai : NHK) for broadcasting. This endoscope enables observation with extreamely low lighting such as LED (Fig. 3) (Kim et al., 2011). We compared conventional endoscopic image with our new endoscopic image to visualize an intrauterine fetal phantom model without the conventinal light source. (Fig. 4). Our new endoscope enabled to visualize the clear fetal face only with a white LED lighting.

2.4 High resolution ultrasound

In current fetus surgery, 3D-ultrasound (3D-US) diagnosis is fundamental to guide endoscopes and surgical instruments. However, the propagation speed of ultrasonic waves are limited so that there is a trade-off between spatial and time resolutions. We developed a high resolution ultrasound apparatus, which includes a new US probe to form transmitting beams simultaneously in two directions and four receiving beams from each transmitting

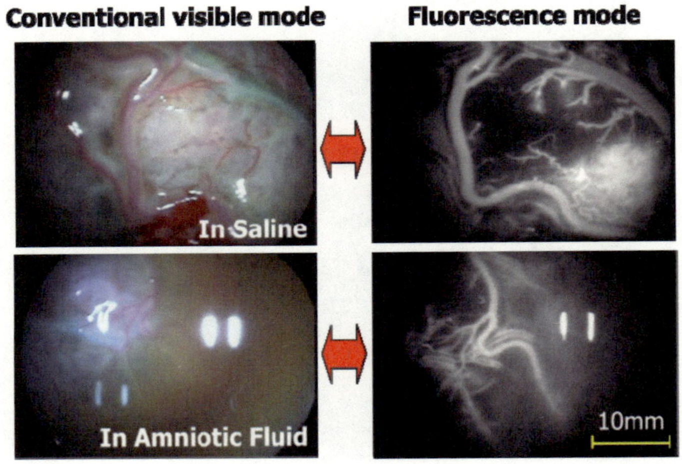

Fig. 2. Fluorescence endoscopic images are visualizing a placenta of cynomolgus monkey. Although the vessels on the placenta are invisible in the cloudy amniotic fluid, they are clearly visible to gain fluorescence from the vessels in the fluorescence mode.

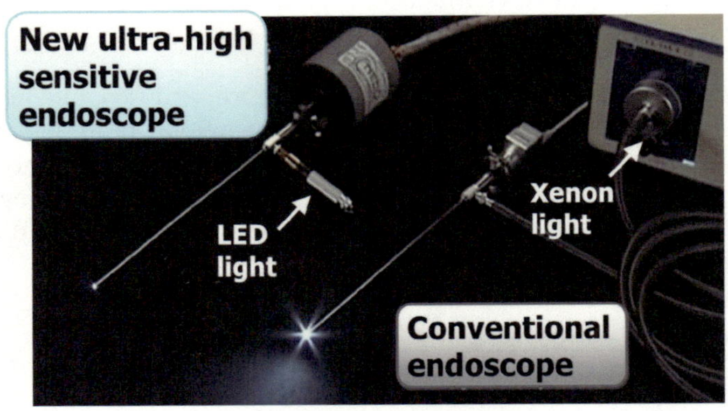

Fig. 3. Appearance of the endoscopes. Left: New ultra-high sensitive endoscope with small LED light. Right: Conventional endoscope with xenon light source.

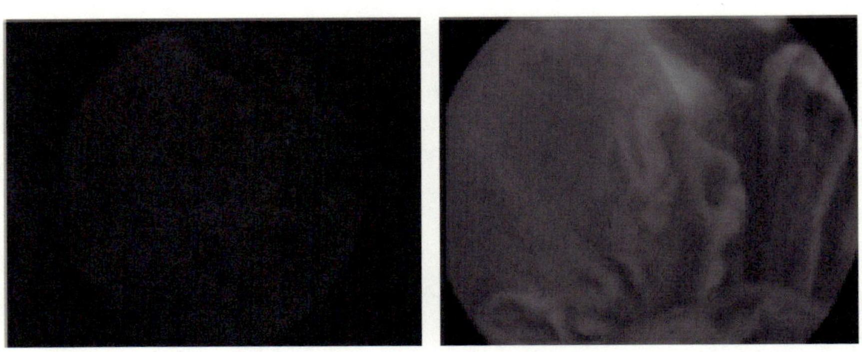

Fig. 4. Comparison of endoscopic image of an intrauterine fetal phantom model without conventional light source. Left: Conventional endoscopic image. Right: New ultra-high sensitive endoscopic image.

beam, to achieve double density volume data in spatial or time resolution (Fig. 5). Using our new apparatus, moving endoscope near intrauterine fetal phantom model are clearly and smoothly visible without diplopia of the endoscope (Fig. 6).

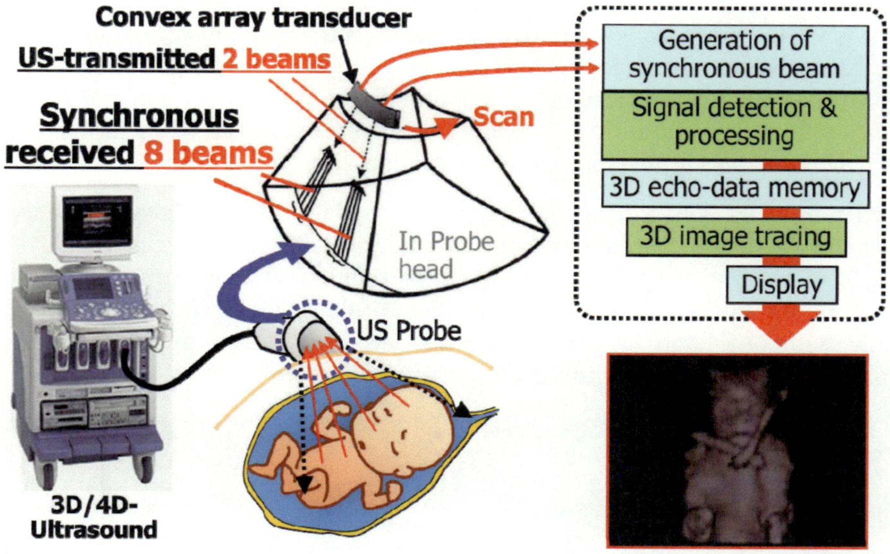

Fig. 5. System configuration of the high resolution ultrasound diagnosis apparatus.

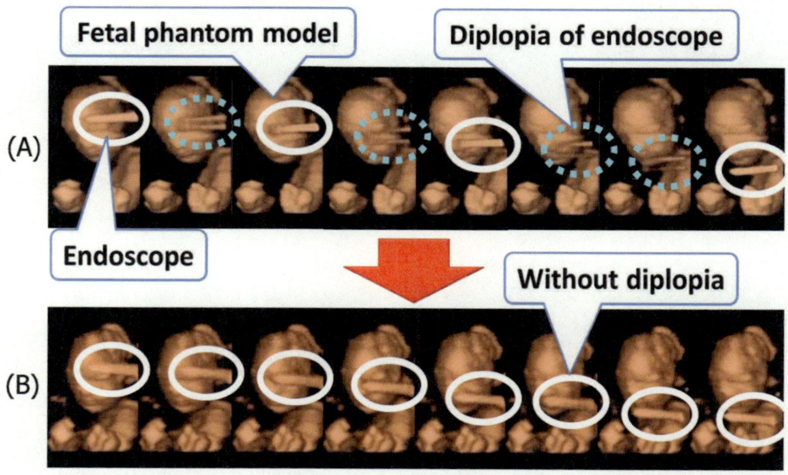

Fig. 6. (A) Conventional 3D-US image including diplopia of the endoscope by frame rate issue. (B) New 3D-US image without diplopia of the endoscope.

3. Super hands

To accomplish a safe and dexterous surgical procedure in utero, we developed specified manipulators (multi degrees-of-freedom) as well as fetal stabilizers having multi-joint distal ends. These devices are 4-mm or less in diameter to minimize uterine injuries and/or reduce perioperative complications.

3.1 Miniature manipulator

Manipulation of surgical instruments in the uterus should be safe, careful and dexterous because of fragile tissues of fetal body, placenta, amniotic membrane and so on. For this issue, we developed two miniature bending manipulators which have multi degrees-of-freedom (DOFs). One is the wire-guided linkage-driven 3.5-mm manipulator with an easily exchangeable distal end-effector such as forceps and laser fiber (Fig. 7: Left) (Yamashita et al., 2008a). The other is the more miniature wire-driven 2.4-mm manipulator (Fig. 7: Right) (Harada et al., 2006). These manipulators are mainly composed of metal (stainless steel, titanium, etc.) and sterilizable for clinical application.

These manipulators with a laser fiber to photocoagulate placental communicating vessels for laser therapy of TTTS were evaluated by underwater phantom or in vitro experiments (Fig. 8), confirming their performance to photo coagulated a wide range of tissues with flexible bending motions. In addition, the 3.5-mm manipulator with forceps is controlled manually with one hand to grasp and pass needle or thread in the intrauterine fetal phantom model dexterously by under endoscopic guidance(Fig. 9).

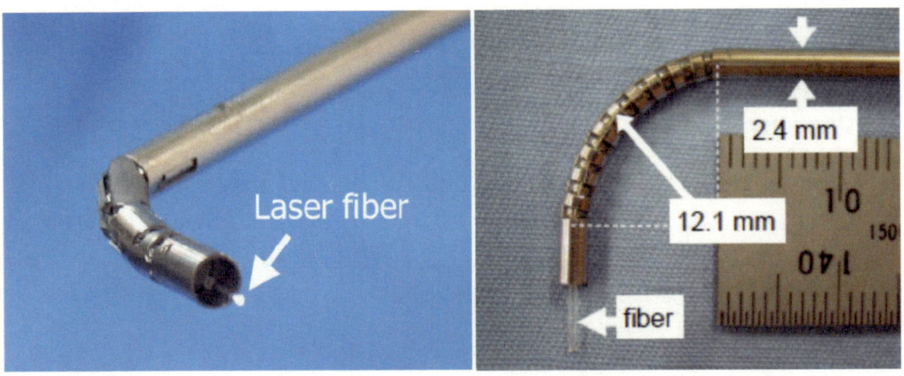

Fig. 7. Distal-end part of the miniature bending laser manipulators with a laser fiber. Left: Wire-guided linkage-driven 3.5-mm manipulator. Right: Wire-driven 2.4-mm manipulator.

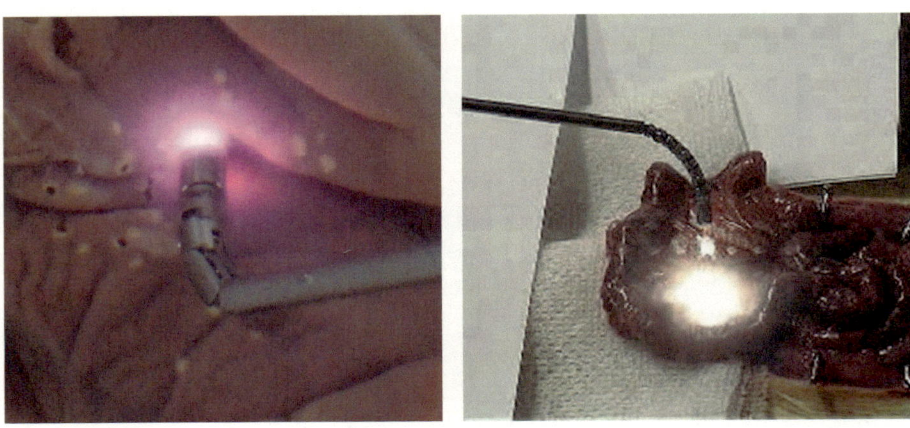

Fig. 8. Left: Nd:YAG laser photocoagulations of the placental phantom model surface with bending motion of the 3.5-mm laser manipulator. Right: Nd:YAG laser photocoagulation of the vessels on the rat mesenterium with the wire-driven 2.4-mm bending laser manipulator.

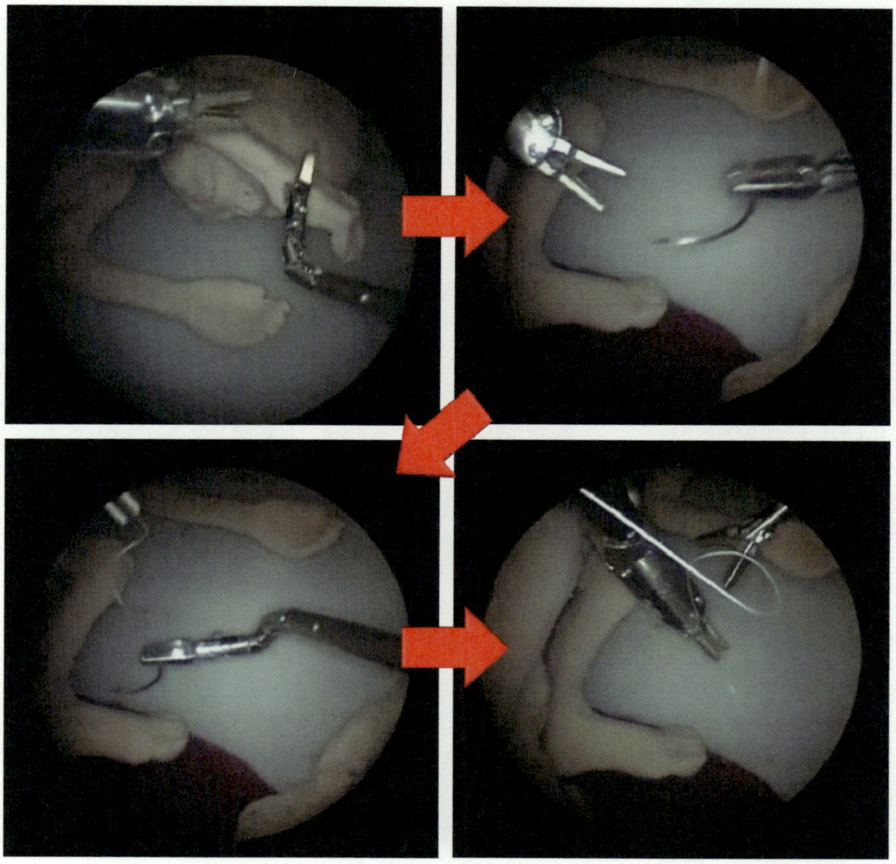

Fig. 9. Bi-manual maneuver evaluation with a new 3.5mm forceps manipulator and previously developed 10-mm forceps manipulator. These manipulators performed transferring a needle or thread endoscopically.

3.2 Bending stabilizer

Safe approach to the intrauterine fetus is difficult because the fetus is floating and rotating in amniotic fluid. For this issue, we developed two types bending stabilizers, especially for the therapy of MMC with a covering patch and laser therapy of TTTS. One is the 2.4-mm wire-driven bending stabilizer to stabilize around the affected area. And the other is the 4-mm wire and linkage-driven balloon manipulator to hold the fetal whole-body softly (Yamanaka et al., 2008). These devices have multi-joints structure and multi-DOFs to approach fetal body non-invasively. We evaluated these devices and confirmed their effective performance in in vitro test with a cynomolgus monkey's brain tissue (Fig. 10: Upper right) and in phantom test with a silicone model (Fig. 10: Under right).

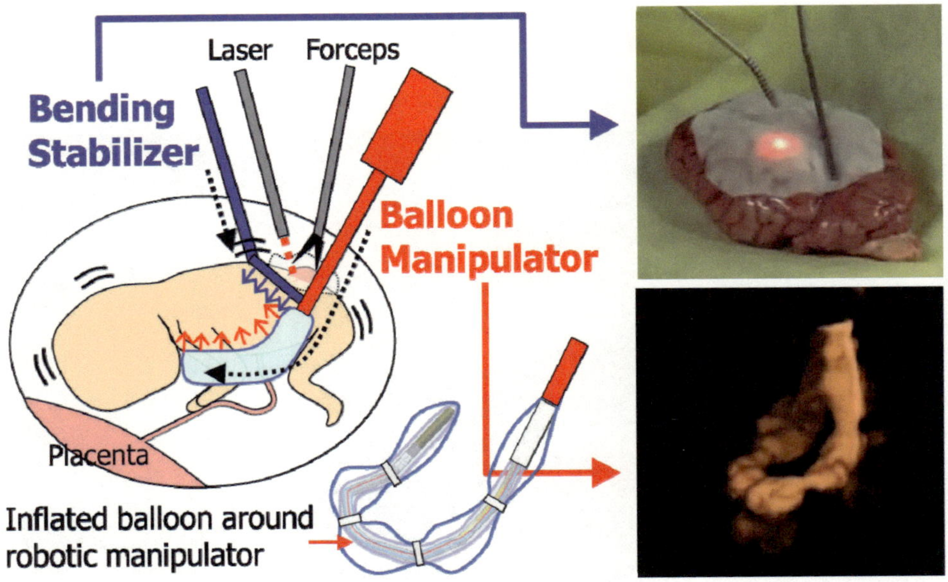

Fig. 10. Bending stabilizer to hold fetal body in uterus. Upper right: In vitro test of the bending stabilizer for laser photocoagulation. Under right: 3D-US image of the bending balloon manipulator in intrauterine phantom model.

4. Combination of "super eye and hands"

To ensure synergy and reduce the number of instruments in use during surgey when separate super eyes and hands are used, We developed two types of super device that comprise super eyes and hands to realize real-time capture of fetoscopic images for effective laser photocoagulation in utero: one is the composite-type laser fiberscope and the other is the computer-aided high-intensity focused ultrasound (HIFU) machine.

4.1 Composite-type laser endoscope

In current laser therapy in fetal surgery, a glass fiber is aligned parallel with a fetoscope, therefore it is difficult to position the laser spot with adequate distance. To solve this problem, we developed two composite-type laser endoscopes. One is the composite-type laser flexible fiberscope including central mono fiber to pass 40-W Yb fiber laser to photocoagulate target tissue with focused energy by a distal-end collective-lens (Fig. 11) (Oka et al., 2010). The outer diameter of this fiberscope is 2.2 mm (Fig. 12), and enables distance measurement with laser Doppler and blood flow detection of targeted blood vessels (Seki et al., 2009, 2010). In *in vivo* test using pig mesenteric vessel underwater, we confirmed occlusion of the vessels by laser photocoagulation fetoscopically (Fig. 13).

The other is a steerable laser endoscope (Yamanaka et al., 2010). Nd: YAG laser from the laser source is reflected by two galvanomirrors in a galvanometer and a beam-splitter to pass through relay lenses in the rigid endoscope. On the other hand, visible light from the distal end of the endoscope passes through the relay lenses and beam-splitter to CCD camera (Fig. 14). The galvanometer is controlled by indication of the laser spot on the

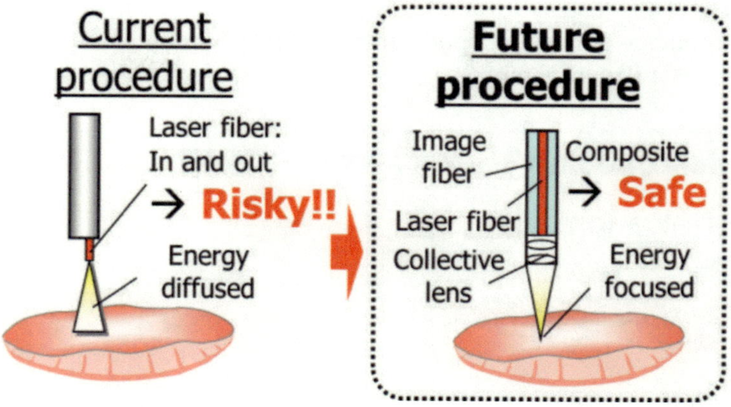

Fig. 11. Concept of the composite-type laser fiberscope.

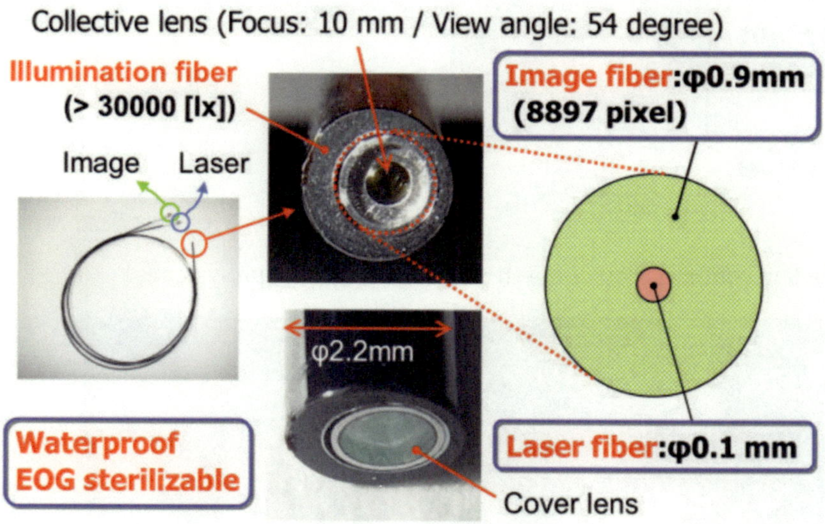

Fig. 12. System configuration of the composite-type laser fiberscope.

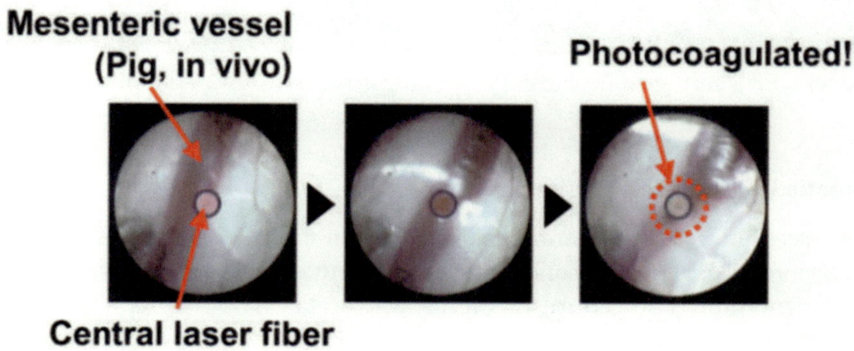

Fig. 13. In vivo test to photocoagulate a mesenteric vessel of swine.

endoscopic view of PC display to steer direction of the Nd:YAG laser beam (Fig. 15). The positioning of accuracy of the laser spot is mostly within 1.0 mm in the endoscopic view at the distance between 10 and 20 mm.

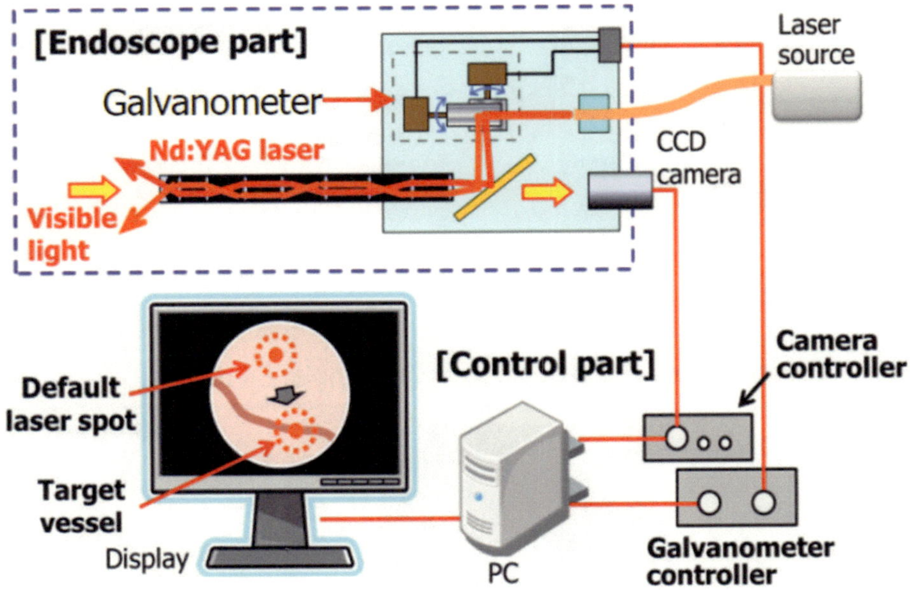

Fig. 14. System configuration of the steerable laser endoscope system.

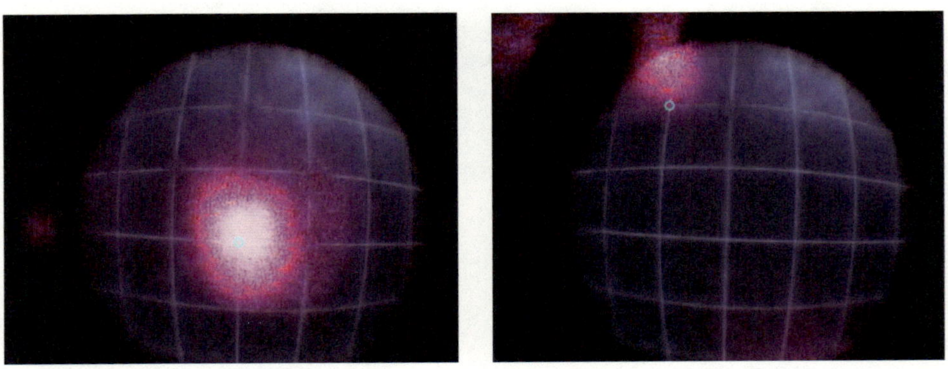

Fig. 15. Laser spot steering control test. Positioning error is around 0.2 mm in the endoscopic view.

4.2 Automatic HIFU delivery system

Current intervention to correct cardiac morphologic abnormalities such as hypoplastic left heart syndrome (HLHS), that is sonographic cardiocentesis for atrioseptostomy is invasive because of penetrating procedure of uterus wall, fetal skin and fetal heart wall. For implementation of minimal invasive cardiac intervention, we take advantage of high intensity focused ultrasound (HIFU), and developed an automatic HIFU delivery system controlled by a real-time computer-based analysis of 2D-US left ventricular images (Fujisaki

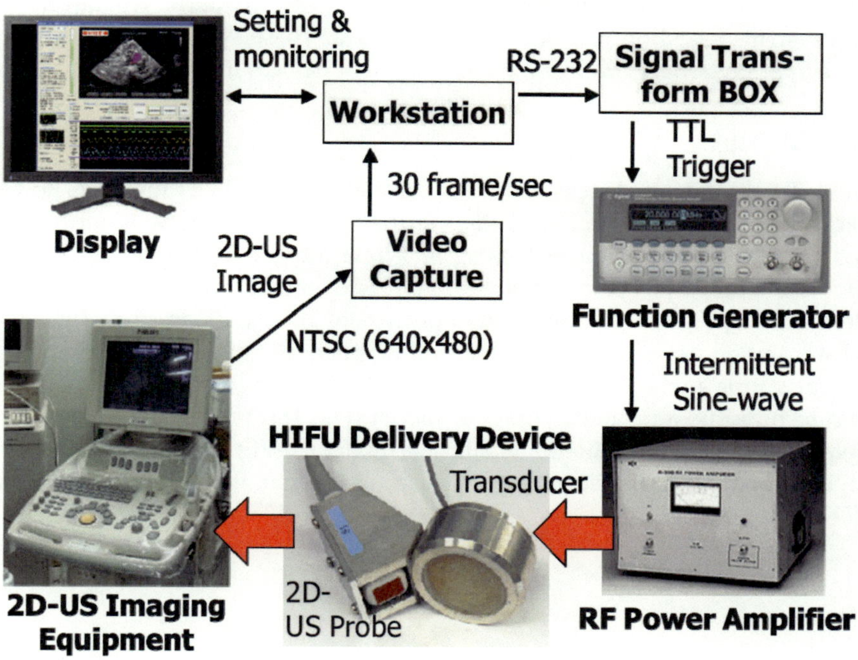

Fig. 16. System configuration of the computer-based automatic HIFU delivery.

et al., 2010; Yamashita et al., 2008b). The system consists of HIFU delivery device with monocoque spherical shaped piezo transducer and diagnostic 2D-US imaging probe, 2D-US imaging equipment, workstation, function generator and RF power amplifier to drive the transducer (Fig. 16). In in vivo evaluation using the beating hearts of anesthetized adult rabbits, the system successfully achieved a non-touch gross ablation and small transmural opening of the atrial septum (Fig. 17).

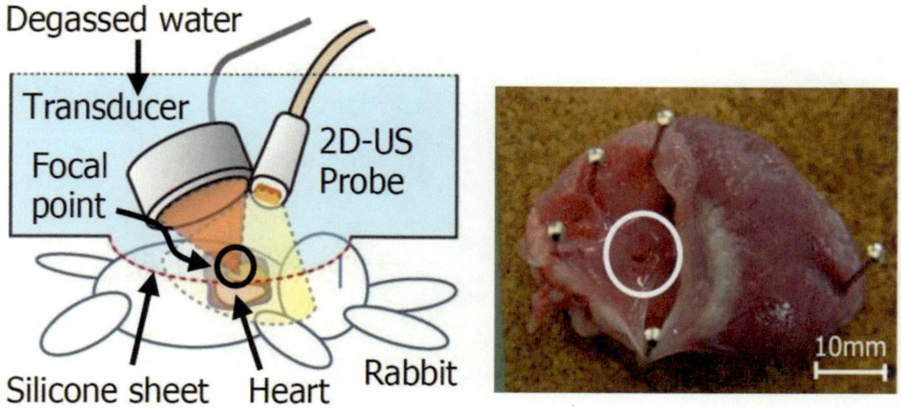

Fig. 17. Experimental setup using an adult rabbit. HIFU delivery was done through a silicone sheet at the bottom of the degassed water tank.

5. Super navigations

To guide surgical devices with much less invasiveness in utero, we developed three navigation systems based on realtime 3D/4D-US data. These systems enable us display of intrauterine operative space for position recognition of devices intuitively.

5.1 On-site 3D display

The current 3D-US data is displayed on 2D dusplay such as LCD monitor, however 3D-image data should be displayed on 3D display from the point of view of intuitiveness. We developed on-site 3D display system using real-time Integral Videography (IV) providing images (or visual display) without any specific glasses unlike general 3D-movie or 3D-TV. Our system can display spatial position and posture of 3D objects precisely by combination of a high-resolution large LCD monitor and a plate of micro-lens array. High-speed computing performs a real-time rendering of 3D-US diagnosis data, and transforms to clear and give a picturesque autostereoscopic 3D-model (Fig. 18). We tested our performance of this system using an intrauterine fetus silicone model, confirming on-site 3D-ultrasaound image of fetus, and surgical instruments from multi-viewpoints with maximum frame rate of 3 Hz (Fig. 19).

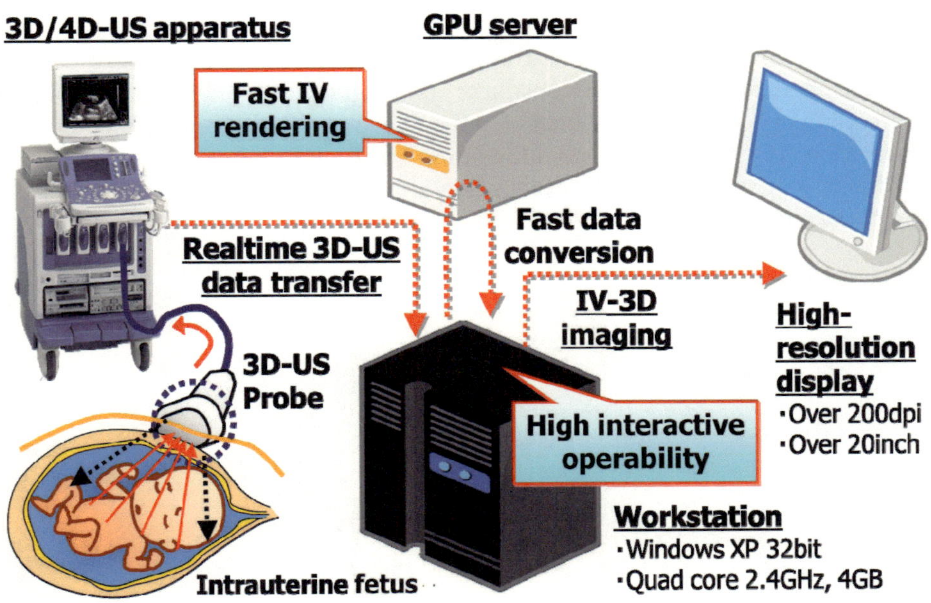

Fig. 18. System configuration of the on-site 3D display with real-time Integral Videography rendering.

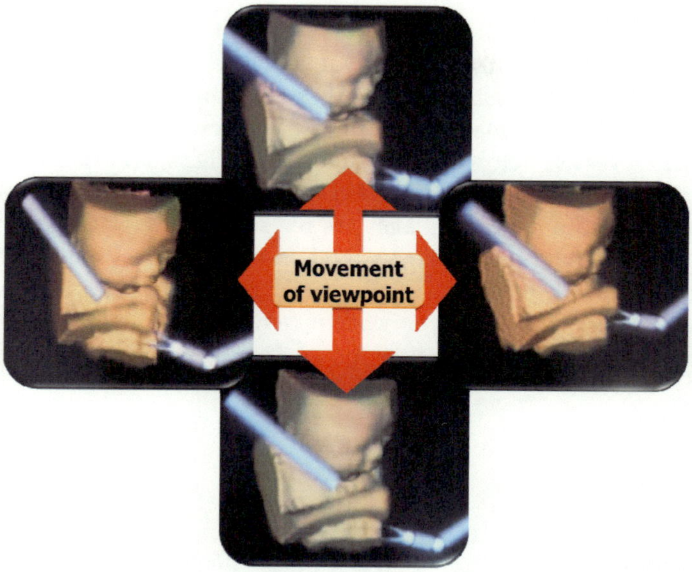

Fig. 19. Feasibility test of the on-site 3D display system to display an intrauterine fetal phantom model with surgical instruments.

5.2 Distance alarm system

The interios of the uterus is very narrow and manipulation of instruments requires the utmost attention. To support the manipulation, we developed a distance alarm system based on a real-time updated 3D/4D-US data. After receiving 3D/4D-US data of uterus and high-speed computing with multi-core processor system, the relative positions of intrauterine tissue and surgical tools such as a fetoscope and feoceps are supplied as a color mapping and warning alarm for surgical navigation (Fig. 20). From the result, accuracy of the system was about 3mm in position error, and the updating time was about 200-500ms.

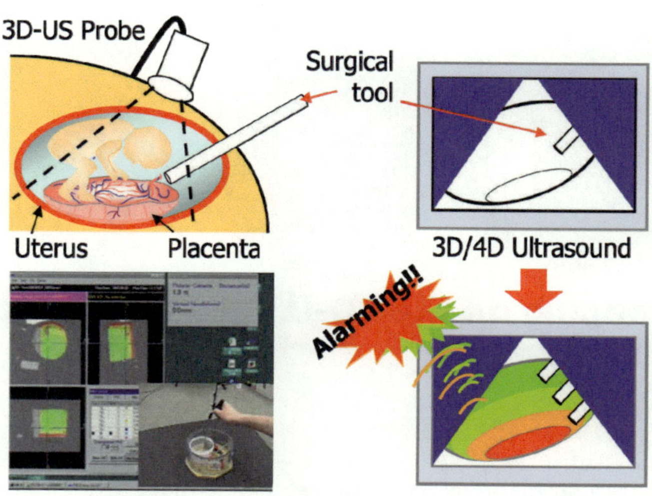

Fig. 20. Color-mapped distance alarming system with alarming caution.

5.3 Placental vascular mapping

In current TTTS laser therapy, the network of placental anastomotic vessels needs to be restructured from the narrow fetoscopic view in the surgeon's head. For this issue, we developed placental vascular mapping system based on the placental 3D-US data and continuous placental vessels' fetoscopic image mosaics (Fig. 21) (Liao et al., 2009). 3D spatial position of the fetoscopic images and the US image are tracked by 3D position tracking device, and the mosaiced fetoscopic images are registered to the surface of 3D-US placenta model by using the fast image rendering method and the seamless multi-images processing. As the fetoscope is moved, the range of placental vessels mapping is enlarged gradually. Results of phantom test show that the system may provide an improved and effrvtive planning and guidance of laser therapy.

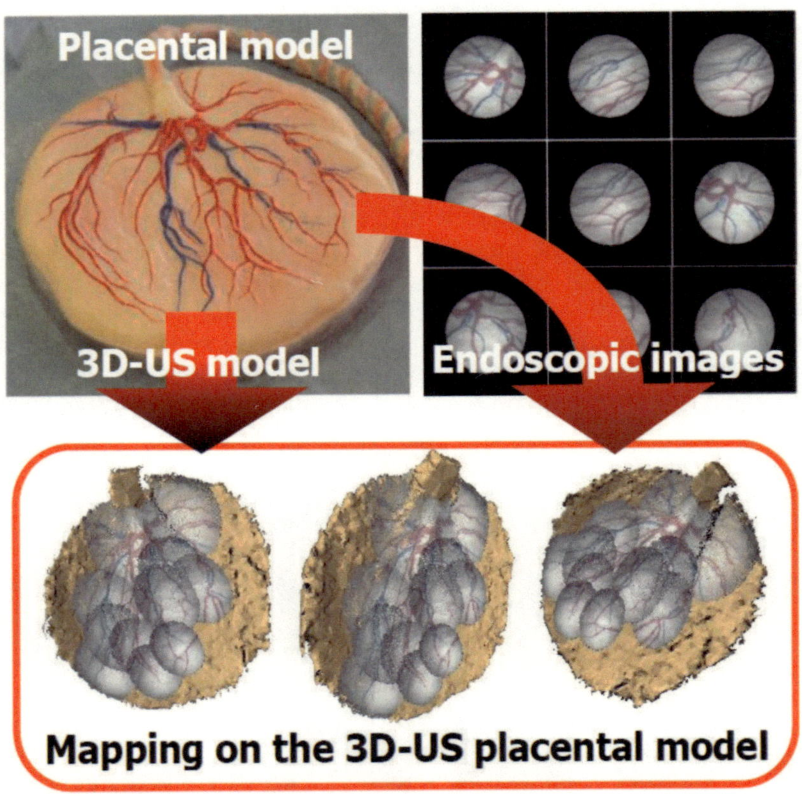

Fig. 21. Placental vascular mapping navigation system to make an entire vessel network by integration of the individual endoscopic images of placenta.

6. Conclusion

Our super devices are certainly useful in future fetal intervention independently. However integration between super eyes, hands and navigations must be more effective surgery, which results in applications in general surgery (Fig. 22). Although part of our device is stil in the experimental phase, there is a device which is ready for a clinical use with high performance. Our research members are making efforts to improve these technologies for future all over the world.

We developed super eyes, hands and navigations of surgeons and these applications for future fetal intervention. These technologies are not only for stand-alone use but also applicable for integrated use. And, because fetal surgery is one of the most difficult surgeries, our achievements will be also applicable to general surgery.

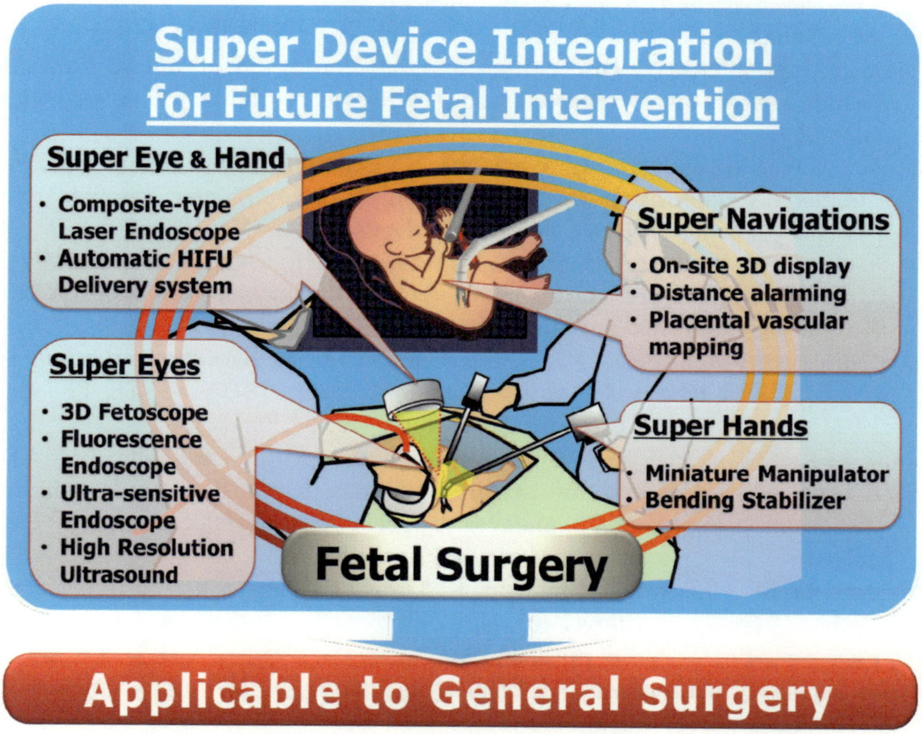

Fig. 22. Overview of super device integration of super eyes, hands and navigations for future fetal intervention, which is applicable to general surgery.

7. Acknowledgement

We wish to thank Akiko Suzuki for help in preparing the manuscript. And a part of this work was supported by Health and Labour Sciences Research Grants (H17-Physi-006, a joint research project among the Ministry of Economy, Trade and Industry, the New Energy and Industrial Technology Development Organization, and the Ministry of Health, Labour, and Welfare (H20-Nano-016), JSPS Grants-in-Aid for Scientific Research (17100008), Research Fellowships of the Japan Society for the Promotion of Science for Young Scientists (041400000227) and Grant Program for Child Health and Development (16-3) administrated by Ministry of Health, Labour and Welfare of Japan.

8. References

Bruner, JP., Richards, WO., Tulipan, NB. & Arney, TL. (1999). Endoscopic coverage of fetal myelomeningocele in utero, *American Journal of Obstetrics and Gynecology*, Vol. 180, Issue 1, pp. 153-158

Feldstein, VA., Machin, GA., Albanese, CT., Sandberg, P., Farrell, JA., Farmer, DL. & Harrison, MR.(2000). Twin-Twin Transfusion Syndrome: The 'Select' Procedure. *Fetal Diagnosis and Therapy*, Vol. 15, No. 5, pp. 257-261

Fujisaki, M., Chiba, T., Enosawa, S., Dohi, T. & Takamoto, S.(2010). Cardiac intervention using high-intensity focused ultrasound: creation of interatrial communication in beating heart of an anesthetized rabbit, *Ultrasound in Obstetrics & Gynecology*, 36(5), 607-612

Harada, K., Miwa, M., Fukuyo, T., Watanabe, S., Enosawa, S. & Chiba, T. (2009). ICG fluorescence endoscope for visualization of the placental vascular network, *Minimally Invasive Therapy & Allied Technologies*, Vol. 18, No. 1, pp. 1-5

Harada, K., Iwase, K., Tsubouchi, K., Kishi, K., Nakamura, T., Chiba, T. & Fujie, MG.(2006). Micro Manipulator and Forceps Navigation for Endoscopic Fetal Surgery, *Journal of Robotics and Mechatronics*, Vol. 18, No. 3, pp. 257-263

Harrison, MR., Evans MI., Adzick, NS. & Holzgreve, W. (2001). *The unborn patient: the art and science of fetal therapy 3rd edition*, Saunders, ISBN 978-0721684468, Philadelphia, USA

Ishiyama, A., Kim, K., Yamashita, H., Miyamoto, Y., Enosawa, S. & Chiba, T.(2011). New fluorescence endoscope for use in twin–twin transfusion syndrome: In vivo visualization of placental blood vessels. *Medical Engineering & Physics*, Vol. 33, pp. 381–385

Kim, K., Kubota, M., Ohkawa, Y., Shiraishi, T., Kawai, T., Kobayashi, A., Yamashita, H. & Chiba, T.(2011). A novel ultralow-illumination endoscope system, *Surgical Endoscopy*, Vol. 25, No. 6, pp. 2029-2033

Kobayashi, E., Ando, T., Yamashita , H., Sakuma, I., Fukuyo, T., Ando, K. & Chiba, T. (2009). A high-resolution, three-dimensional thin endoscope for fetal surgery, *Surgical Endoscopy*, Vol. 23, No. 11, pp. 2450-2453

Kohl, T., Hering, R., Heep, A., Schaller, C., Meyer, B., Greive, C., Bizjak, G., Buller, T., van de Vondel, P., Gogarten, W., Bartmann, P., Knöpfle, G. & Gembruch, U. (2006). Percutaneous Fetoscopic Patch Coverage of Spina Bifida Aperta in the Human - Early Clinical Experience and Potentioal, *Fetal Diagnosis and Therapy*, Vol. 21, No. 2, pp. 185-193

Kohl, T., Sharland, G., Allan, LD., Gembruch, U., Chaoui, R., Lopes, LM., Zielinsky, P., Huhta, J. & Silverman, NH.(2000). World experience of percutaneous ultrasound-guided balloon valvuloplasty in human fetuses with severe aortic valve obstruction. *The American Journal of Cardiology*, Vol. 85, Issue 10, pp. 1230-1233

Liao, H., Tsuzuki, M., Mochizuki, T., Kobayashi, E., Chiba, T. & Sakuma, I.(2009). Fast image mapping of endoscopic image mosaics with three-dimensional ultrasound image for intrauterine fetal surgery, *Minimally Invasive Therapy & Allied Technologies*, Vol. 18, No. 3, pp. 32–34

Marshall, AC., van der Velde, ME., Tworetzky, W., Gomez, CA., Wilkins-Haug, L., Benson, CB., Jennings, RW. & Lock, JE.(2004). Creation of an atrial septal defect in utero for fetuses with hypoplastic left heart syndrome and intact or highly restrictive atrial septum. Circulation, Vol. 110, Issue 3, pp. 253-258

Mäkikallio, K., McElhinney, DB., Levine, JC., Marx, GR., Colan, SD., Marshall, AC., Lock, JE., Marcus, EN. & Tworetzky, W.(2006). Fetal Aortic valve stenosis and the evolution of hypoplastic left heart syndrome patient selection for fetal intervention, Circulation, Vol. 113, pp. 1401-1405

Oka, K., Seki, T., Naganawa, A., Yamashita, H., Kim, K. & Chiba, T.(2010). The development of composite-type optical fiberscope system for fetoscopic laser photocoagulation of chorionic plate anastomosing vessels (FLPC), *Minimally Invasive Therapy & Allied Technologies*, Vol. 19, No. 2, pp. 94-99

Quintero, RA., Comas, C., Bornick, PW., Allen, MH. & Kruger, M.(2000). Selective versus non-selective laser photocoagulation of placental vessels in twin-to-twin transfusion syndrome, *Ultrasound Obsted Gynecoogyl*, Vol. 16, Issue 3, pp. 230-236

Seki, T., Oka, K., Naganawa, A., Yamashita, H., Kim, K., Chiba, T.(2010). Laser distance measurement using a newly developed composite-type optical fiberscope for fetoscopic laser surgery, *Optics and Lasers in Engineering*, Vol. 48, pp. 974–97

Seki, T., Oka, K., Naganawa, A., Yamashita, H., Kim, K. & Chiba, T.(2009). Blood flow measurement system for fetoscopic laser photocoagulation of chorionic plate anastomosing vessels, *Minimally Invasive Therapy & Allied Technologies*, Vo. 18, No. 6, pp. 350-355

Senat, MV., Deprest, Jan., Boulvain, M., Paupe, A., Winer, N. & Ville, Y.(2004). Endoscopic Laser Surgery versus Serial Amnioreduction for Severe Twin-to-Twin Transfusion Syndrome. *The New England Journal of Medicine*, Vol. 351, Issue 2, pp. 136-144

Yamanaka, N., Yamashita, H., Masamune, K., Chiba, T. & Dohi, T.(2010). An endoscope with 2 DOFs steering of coaxial Nd:YAG laser beam for fetal surgery. Mechatronics, IEEE/ASME Transactions on Mechatoronics, Vol. 15, Issue. 6, pp. 898-905

Yamanaka, N., Yamashita, H., Matsumiya, K., Liao, H., Masamune, K., Chiba, T. & Dohi, T.(2008). Surgical Manipulator with Balloon for Stabilizing Fetus in Utero under Ultrasound Guidance, *Proceedings of Medical Imaging and Augmented Reality 4th International Workshop (MIAR2008)*, Lecture Notes in Computer Science (LNCS) 5128, pp. 260-269, Tokyo, Japan, July 2008

Yamashita, H., Matsumiya, K., Masamune, K., Liao, H., Chiba, T. & Dohi, T.(2008a) Miniature bending manipulator for fetoscopic intrauterine laser therapy in twin-to-twin transfusion syndrome, *Surgical Endoscopy*, Vol. 22, No. 2, pp. 430-435

Yamashita, H., Ishii, T., Ishiyama, A., Nakayama, N., Miyoshi, T., Miyamoto, Y., Kitazumi, G., Katsuike, Y., Okazaki, M., Azuma, T., Fujisaki, M., Takamoto, S., Chiba, T.(2008b). Computer-aided Delivery of High-Intensity Focused Ultrasound (HIFU) for Creation of an Atrial Septal Defect In vivo, *Proceedings of Medical Imaging and Augmented Reality 4th International Workshop (MIAR2008),* Lecture Notes in Computer Science (LNCS) 5128, pp. 300-310, Tokyo, Japan, July 2008